God Needs Me

God Needs Me
living with dysautonomia

LYNN FOX ADAMS

Tate Publishing & Enterprises

Published by Tate Publishing & Enterprises, LLC
127 E. Trade Center Terrace | Mustang, Oklahoma 73064 USA
1.888.361.9473 | www.tatepublishing.com

Tate Publishing is committed to excellence in the publishing industry. The company reflects the philosophy established by the founders, based on Psalm 68:11,
"The Lord gave the word and great was the company of those who published it."

Book design copyright © 2009 by Tate Publishing, LLC. All rights reserved.
Cover design by Kellie Southerland
Interior design by Stefanie Rooney

Published in the United States of America

ISBN: 978-1-60799-592-0
1. Medical, Diseases
2. Religion, Christian Life, Inspirational
09.06.26

Dedication

This book is lovingly dedicated to my mother-in-law, Opal W. Adams (1932–1997). She was full of compassion and love for all people. Everyone who knew her loved her. She was my best friend and one that I could admire. I am eternally grateful for the life lessons she taught me. Although I was sick most of the years we shared, she would say, "I accept you. I think I will keep you around."

To my husband, Ken, the man who has taught me what love is; thank you for never giving up on me when others did. Thank you for believing in me no matter what. You amaze me more and more every day by your hard work and the passion you have for the First Baptist Church of Opelika. Your unconditional love has helped mold me into the person I am today.

To Tricia and Kenneth, my two children; you both have brought joy and meaning to my life. Being your mom has been my greatest reward.

This book is also dedicated to Dr. Cecil Coughlin. He is a remarkable man who has given decades of his life to helping people with dysautonomia. He is to be commended and honored because he has given so many people around the world hope when they needed it most.

Finally, this book is dedicated to the people who make up the First Baptist Church of Opelika for your love, loyalty, support, acceptance, and help. So many of you have shown me what love really is. Thank you, Reverend Scoggins, for every visit to the hospital and for the many candy bars and prayers. You are a wonderful, caring pastor who shares Jesus's love by your actions.

Acknowledgments

I would like to thank Dr. Ross Davis for his dedication to go where no doctor has gone before and to his whole staff for getting me out of the nursing home. Thanks especially to his nurses, Carolyn, Lynn, and Tim, for putting up with my many calls for help and for their patience and the help they have given me throughout the years.

I can't forget the intensive care unit at East Alabama Medical Center for helping me get on the drug Levophed. It took a group effort of three long months. Thanks also to the team of doctors who helped me when I had a deadly infection in 2008.

A special thank you to Mrs. Libba Prochaska, who was my Girl Scout leader for ten years. She taught me so many survival skills that I still use today.

H & M Drugs has been fantastic to supply me with whatever intravenous drugs I needed. They have also been great moral support. Thanks to all of you.

The people in my community have been wonderful. My appreciation goes to Holy Trinity Episcopal Church for helping my children through college by giving them a book scholarship every year.

My next-door neighbor, Wanda Duck, is such a great example of what a neighbor should be. She shows her love through actions and brings me food when I can't get up and comes over when I need IV fluids. She has even worked in our yard. I cannot thank her enough for her thoughtfulness. She is a wonderful neighbor and one to be admired.

I am thankful to Pepperell Baptist Church for your support and prayers.

Thank you to the ladies from First Baptist who walked around the fountain and prayed for me every day for weeks. Your prayers were greatly felt and appreciated.

Thank you to a friend for helping me edit this book.

I especially want to thank Marie and Woody Tully for the computer they supplied to me so I could write this book. You both are amazing. Thank you, Marie, for stepping in as my adoptive mom. I love you.

Especially, I am humbled by what God has done in my life for his glory—not mine. Thank you, my awesome God.

Table of Contents

Foreword

It is estimated that more than one million Americans suffer from the various forms of dysautonomia. The autonomic nervous system (ANS) controls and regulates all of the body's involuntary actions, such as respiration, blood pressure, heart rate, digestion, and many other vital functions necessary to maintain life. Any disease or illness that impairs these functions is known as dysautonomia.

In 1997 we established the National Dysautonomia Research Foundation (NDRF). Our mission was to provide patients with both information and support. One area that was in desperate need of help was patient support. Soon after we placed an announcement online that we were looking for volunteers to assist in our mission, we heard from a young woman named Lynn Adams.

Lynn was a happy and outgoing individual who wanted to help. Lynn suffered from dysautonomia. Although it was not unusual for us to hear from patients who wanted to volunteer or assist, what was highly unusual was that Lynn was completely bedridden in a nursing home.

Uncertain that Lynn could physically contribute, I suggested she run the support group from her hometown of Opelika, Alabama. Believing that Lynn would only last a week or two, I was unprepared for what came next. Lynn did something no one else did. She got on the phone and started to call her state senators and congressmen. She also made calls to her local Elk's and Lion's Club, raising an amazing $5,000. All of Lynn's calls were made from her bed in a quiet and lonely nursing home. I still remember speaking with Lynn and overhearing her nurses inform her that she needed to rest.

By the end of the first year, Lynn had raised more than $7,500 to help support our mission. To recognize Lynn's efforts, we awarded her the Presidential Volunteer Award in Washington, DC. While in Washington, Lynn boarded a Campus Hill Police Bus and testified before members of both the House and Senate as well as members of the Senate Health Committee, on the devastating impact that dysautonomia has on its patients and our country.

The stressful day caused Lynn to become seriously ill. Fortunately an expert on dysautonomia was summoned to her hotel room, where help was given. Lynn was then flown home, assisted by her personal physician and nurse. While in flight, Lynn once again became violently ill. The event nearly cost Lynn her life.

Unmoved by the fact that her body was working against her, Lynn has continued to fight this disease process. Her incredible faith in Christ is inspiring. Regardless of how Lynn is feeling, she will always greet you with a smile and a joyous, cheerful heart. Lynn's love for God has most certainly made her the perfect support group leader. In fact, Lynn now coordinates support groups throughout the U.S. and

Canada on our online website. More than twenty thousand members each month benefit from Lynn's compassion. To me, it is obvious that Lynn is walking in the Lord's footsteps. Or maybe it is the Lord who continues to lift her to miraculous heights.

Linda J. Smith
Founder/Executive Director
National Dysautonomia Research
Foundation (NDRF)

Introduction

We have been sent to speak for Christ.

2 Corinthians 5:20, NIV

When I came to you, I was weak and fearful and trembling.

1 Corinthians 2:3, NIV

My life is worth nothing unless I use it for doing the work assigned to me by the Lord Jesus—the work of telling others the good news about God's wonderful kindness and love.

Acts 20:24, NIV

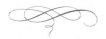

This true story is full of twists and turns that will keep you on the edge of your seat. While you flip through the pages and read the miracles God has performed, you will be amazed. I was able to write this book with the help of journal entries and newspaper articles.

The title of the book comes from working for God. So many times we say, "I need you, Lord." But really God needs us here on earth to share the gospel and his love.

Although I speak of painful times with my family, I pray that this book will not be hurtful to them. The events I speak of are truthful. It is my prayer that my relatives who have disowned me will some-day come to terms with it.

I pray God will use this book to help others learn how to cope with dysautonomia or any other chronic illness by putting God first in their lives.

Despite the overwhelming odds, I, my husband, Ken, and our two kids have overcome this illness. That doesn't mean things are easy. They are actually difficult, but if we continue to lean on God, we can stay strong. Ken and I have proven that you can raise your children to be strong Christians, even if one parent has a chronic illness. Even if you suffer from a physical condition, you can constantly pray for your family members. As I look back, I can see a reason for every tear I have shed and for every pain I have felt. God used my circumstances to improve my spiritual life and help others with similar conditions.

It is my prayer that, through this book, you will learn how to live with dysautonomia. I cannot imagine suffering without God by my side. If you do not suffer from dysautonomia, it is my prayer that you will understand the difficulties people have living with this condition or other debilitating diseases.

·

Finding a Doctor

So many times, you go see a doctor, but if he is not trained on the autonomic function of the body (dys-autonomia), then he cannot help you. I too went to several doctors before I finally got the right diagnosis. In this book, you will read about my struggles of finding a doctor. The one I have now is intelligent, caring, and giving, and understands the autonomic nervous system.

Some of you have lost relationships with family members because of your illness. I too have lost family due to the fact that they do not believe I am sick. You will see my struggles to try and make my family understand and accept me. If you have lost family members, do not forget that God loves you more than anyone ever can. He also accepts you the way you are, and his love is unconditional.

·

Chronic Condition

It doesn't matter which chronic condition you suffer from; you too can live a life filled with peace, joy, and love through Jesus Christ our Lord. This book is filled with times God used my life while I was chronically ill. Not having a break from our condition makes us struggle the most. Dr. Ross Davis told me one time, "Your good day is a normal person's bad day." I have found that that quote is so true.

Totally Bedridden

There were times when I was so sick that I couldn't get out of bed. From the years 1994 to 1999, I was totally bedridden in my room in our house. I was actually trapped, unable to sit up without passing out. This book will tell you how I handled that. I was amazed at what God did through me while I was lying flat on my back. God used my condition for his glory.

God can use you also if you have a personal relationship with him. You can comfort others the same way you have been comforted through Jesus Christ. Keep in mind that Jesus suffered too.

You are not alone. Many people who suffer from dysautonomia feel alone and unaccepted. I felt that way many times. Read how God showed me that I was loved and accepted by him. You need to give it all to the Lord.

Florida

I grew up in sunny Florida. I can remember going to the beach with my friends. While they lay in the sun getting tans, I could not. It made me feel sick, dizzy, and tired, so I swam while they tanned. I passed out several times throughout my life when I was young but just didn't know why. I knew my body was fighting something. I later found out it was dysautonomia.

I was very active, rode my bike, swam, and sat on the beach in the evenings when it was cooler. On the corner of my street was a Baptist church. I thank God for that church. That was where I learned how to live for the Lord. Many adults in the church inspired me and helped me live for Jesus Christ. I attended every time the doors were open. Some of my friends had dads who were deacons. As I spent time with them at their homes, I learned what it was like to live a godly life. I learned so much from the Nolands and the Tisdales. Acteens taught me how to minister to others. My leader, Mrs. Littleston, taught me how to be a missionary; she has a special place in my heart. As part of Acteens, we visited the nursing homes often. Little did I know, I would end up living in one at the age of thirty-seven. You will read stories of how God gave me peace, joy, and love while I was in the nursing home. It was amazing what God did through my life while I was flat on my back. God can use you too.

Miracles

Miracles come in all types: physical, mental, and spiritual. Throughout this book, you will read about the miracles God has performed in my life. Whether sick or well, we are here on earth for God, not ourselves. You will learn that all you need to get through the difficult days is God. Sit back and read about God's wondrous and mighty plan.

What Is Dysautonomia?

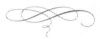

Dysautonomia is the condition caused by a malfunction of the autonomic nervous system (ANS), a part of the body's nervous system. There are many different ways the autonomic system can be disrupted; therefore, there are many disorders resulting from such malfunctions.

The body's internal organs—such as the heart, stomach, and intestines—are all regulated by the ANS. The ANS is a part of the peripheral nervous system, whose functions are involuntary or reflexive. For example, we do not have control over our blood vessels or when our hearts beat faster.

The ANS manages the body's complex tasks to maintain a stable internal condition and responds to changes that take place in our external surroundings. Examples include when the external temperature causes us to sweat, lowering our internal temperature, and when an intense situation causes a fight-or-flight reaction. Heart rate and blood pressure allow us to cope and reverse these actions when the situation has resolved. Some things that can affect the ANS are hot weather, temperature changes, posture, food intake, change, stress, and emotional situations. Imagine what can happen if the ANS is so out of balance that even food intake and posture can affect it.

Since the autonomic nervous system manages most of the bodily systems—the cardiovascular system, gastrointestinal, urinary and bowel functions, temperature regulation, reproduction, and our metabolic and endocrine systems—it can be very difficult to describe how it works.

The autonomic nervous system sends messages to the appropriate end organs (heart, blood vessels, stomach) by releasing transmitter substances to which the receptors of the target cells are responsive. The ANS conveys sensory impulses from the blood vessels, the heart, and all of the organs in the chest, abdomen, and pelvis through nerves to the other parts of the brain. These impulses do not reach our consciousness but instead initiate autonomic, or reflex, responses through the efferent nerves. This causes the appropriate reaction of the heart, the vascular system, and all the organs of the body to any variations in our environment.

It is estimated that more than five hundred thousand Americans are afflicted with this type of dysautonomia, which is orthostatic intolerance. It is found predominantly in women. The onset can be sudden and can have a severe impact on the person. It often leaves young women unable to work or care for their small children. Often these conditions tend to be misdiagnosed as depression or anxiety disorders due to the similar symptoms. Misunderstanding by their doctors tends to lead to a misunderstanding in their families, resulting in the loss of relationships and broken homes and often friends, leaving many alone and desperately needing help.

Standing upright results in a series of reflexive bodily responses regulated by the autonomic nervous system to compensate for the effect of gravity upon the distribution of blood. The normal response for a change in body position results in stabilization to the upright position in approximately sixty seconds. The normal change in heart rate would include an increased heart rate of ten to fifteen beats per minute and an increase in diastolic pressure of 10mm Hg with only a slight change in systolic pressure. For those who are afflicted with orthostatic intolerant dysautonomia, there is an excessive increase in heart rate upon standing, resulting in the cardiovascular system working harder to maintain blood pressure and blood flow to the brain. This often causes passing out or nearly passing out.

Living with Dysautonomia

Living with dysautonomia is very difficult. It is a condition that is hard to understand and very hard to control. Due to its symptoms, some doctors misdiagnose the disease as anxiety or depression issues. The thing is, some people who suffer from dysautonomia *do* have depression and anxiety as well. They fight depression because they have dysautonomia and are often not accepted or have become isolated. Most of us have a lot of stress because of the condition. What has been painful to me is the fact that my own relatives do not believe me. They do not even think I *am* ill. I currently have the support of my husband, Ken, my daughter, Tricia, and my son, Kenneth, and also a cousin, one uncle, and one aunt. But as far as the rest of my family is concerned, no one believes me.

I want those who suffer from dysautonomia to learn through this book how to feel loved, even without the help of family members. One day years ago, someone had to pave a way for cancer treatments. Over the last decade, as I have e-mailed and spoken to people who suffer from dysautonomia, I have noticed that approximately 65 percent of these people are not accepted by their relatives and friends. People do lose connections and the support of family members at times due to an illness. I never thought that would happen to me, but it did. I needed them to say, "I am here for you. It will be okay. We love you." Instead, I was told, "Get up. Get over it , and stop acting sick." Those words were always so painful.

I am so thankful God sent me a doctor who is willing to learn about the condition and do research. In this chapter and the next two, you will read my struggles on finding the right doctor. It is so good finally to have a smart, caring doctor who knows about my physical condition and accepts me. This means so much to me because of the rejection I have felt from some of my own family. But God accepts and loves me. He accepts and loves you too.

"Praise is to the God and Father of our Lord Jesus Christ the Father of compassion and the God of all comfort" (2 Corinthians 1:3, NIV). The verse states "in all comfort;" not just some, but all. You just have to let God in so he can comfort you. He won't give up on you like humans do. God has so much compassion. I have felt it on my worst days. God has helped me learn how to cope while living with dysautonomia.

"Who comforts us in all our troubles, so that we

can comfort those in any trouble with the comfort we ourselves have received from God" (2 Corinthians 1:4, NIV). There it is again. He comforts us in *all* our troubles, not just one certain trouble. Throughout my illness God has comforted me through his Word and through music. When I spent time with him was when I felt his comfort.

"Freely you have received; freely give" (Matthew 10:8, NIV). I am giving you the same comfort I have received. Give it all to God—not some things, all things—because God will help you in all of your troubles.

"For just as the sufferings of Christ flow over into our lives, so also through Christ our comfort overflows" (2 Corinthians 1:5, NIV). This verse states that the suffering of Christ flows into our lives. That is so true; Jesus died on the cross for us to save us from our sins. God's comfort can be shared to help others with the same help you have received. You can have comfort through Jesus Christ, our Lord. Just try it. It really works.

"If we are distressed, it is for your comfort and salvation; if we are comforted, it is for your comfort, which produces in you patient endurance of the same sufferings we suffer" (2 Corinthians 1:6, NIV). Think about it. If we never got distressed, we would never appreciate the fact that it draws us closer to God. If I had never gotten sick, I wouldn't have helped others who suffer from dysautonomia. And the joy of helping others is so awesome. You know, sometimes stress is for our comfort because you then endure the same sufferings as Christ. Being sick can actually make you a stronger person.

"And our hope for you is firm, because we know that just as you share in our sufferings, so also you share in our comfort" (2 Corinthians 1:7, NIV). *Those in Christ will be comforted.* It doesn't say those who *aren't* in Christ will be comforted. This is why it is so important to have a relationship with God. I found comfort in God; miracles happened spiritually, physically, and mentally. I leaned totally on God, and he comforted me through all the troubling times. Jesus Christ died for our sins and rose again. If we believe, we will be comforted. If saved, we will go to heaven when we die on earth.

I started a support group for the National Dysautonomia Research Foundation. Over the years, I have talked to and e-mailed at least several thousand people who needed support. I spent endless hours e-mailing and writing those desperate people. I kept hearing the same thing over and over: doctors telling their patients that it is all in their heads, making family members doubt their loved ones instead of loving and supporting them. They end up with feelings of neglect and sometimes even begin doubting themselves. For years, I tried to pretend to be well because my family didn't accept my illness. That was wrong. I am made perfect because God made me, and he doesn't make mistakes.

"Before I formed you in the womb I knew you, before you were born I set you apart" (Jeremiah 1:5, NIV). We need to remember this scripture, especially if we are feeling unaccepted. God accepted us. He formed us in our mothers' wombs, and he already knew us and loved us. Don't feel bad or guilty about being sick. God can use you if you let him.

"For we are God's workmanship, created in Christ Jesus to do good works, which God prepared in advance for us to do" (Ephesians 2:10, NIV). You see, God prepared us to do good works, and he did it in advance. He knows what good works he has planned for us. I didn't realize that until I became sick. Then I leaned on God. It was then that God started using my life to witness to others. It was in his plan all along.

Things started to get worse physically in 1989. I worked on the Auburn University campus at the Auburn University Federal Credit Union as a supervisor. I worked all day, and on my drive home every day I started to feel so ill that I would have to pull off the road before I passed out. I barely made it home each day. Several times at work, I had to go into the restroom and lie on the floor until I recovered. I even passed out in the line at the grocery store. The scary thing was that I had my son, who was only five years old, with me. I was so blessed no one took him.

On another day, after blacking out, I left work to see my physician. He said, "You are tired and overworked. Go home and rest for four days." He thought maybe it was an inner ear problem. When I went back to see him, he sent me to the emergency room for the help he couldn't give me. I was then sent to see a cardiologist.

The cardiologist ran numerous tests and EP studies, and I was told I had ventricular tachycardia, a serious heart condition. I was put on a heart medication so strong that I couldn't function. I felt guilty about missing so much work and not being able to take care of my family, but I was unable to do anything about it. I continued to struggle from 1989 until 1992.

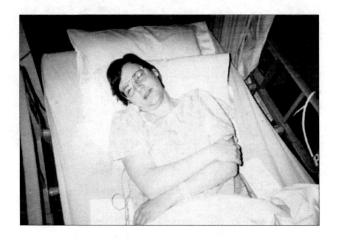

In 1992 I was sent to a cardiologist in Birmingham, Dr. Little. He ran several tests also. He said, "You have dysautonomia, not ventricular tachycardia." That was the first time I had heard of it. The next couple of years were very difficult. I tried to keep up with my job, my family, and my church, but it seemed impossible. I would pick my kids up from the sitters and barely make it home. One day, my daughter was getting in the car, and I drove off while she only had her foot in the door. She was lying in the street but was unharmed. I was in a hurry to get home due to my condition; I didn't want to pass out. I sometimes spent days passed out and often crawled from place to place to avoid hurting myself.

As I mentioned, dysautonomia is a chronic condition. When you suffer from a chronic condition, you do not get a break. It would be like running a race that never ends. You have to continue to run for years and be constantly exhausted. That is what it is like for so many of us who suffer chronically. I began to learn that the only time I felt like I had a break was when I helped others and got my mind off of myself while sharing God's Word.

I had always put my hope in doctors. I used to think they knew everything, but they are not trained on every condition. So I learned to put my hope in God. Yes, I needed a doctor, but I had to pray about it and find the right one.

> This is what the Lord says, "Cursed is the one who trusts in man, who depends on flesh for his strength and whose heart turns away from the Lord. He will be like a bush in the wastelands; he will dwell in the parched places of the desert, in a salt land where no one lives.
> Jeremiah 17:5–6, NIV

Many times, people with an illness put all their hope in doctors when they should put their hope in God. Yes, you need doctors, but how many times have you been anticipating seeing a doctor only to hear, "I can't help you," or, "It's all in your head"?

God knows all and is the great physician. Do not turn your heart against him. Seek help from doctors, but put most of your hope in God, for he is stronger. The fact is, whether sick or well, we are here on earth because of God—to love one another and share his love. That is when you can feel God's peace, joy, and love.

I have a saying: "I am bad physically and at times bad emotionally, but good spiritually, so I am winning the battle."

JOURNAL ENTRY

Dear Lord,

Living with dysautonomia is impossible at times. It affects so many of my bodily functions. Please help me find the proper help I need. I also need my family to love and believe in me. I pray for the right doctor to help me and for one who can help all the thousands who do not have physicians trained on the condition. I am putting my hope in you. I need you, Lord, along with so many others. Help me, even in the midst of illness, learn how to have your peace, joy, and love. Help me reach out to others.

Lynn

A New Doctor and the Tilt Table Test

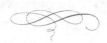

Since I had two different opinions, in 1994 I sought out a specialist for dysautonomia. Once I found him, I wrote a letter begging him to see me, and he agreed. Ken and I flew out. I could barely handle the flight. If it hadn't been for Ken's support, I wouldn't have made it. I laid my head on him the whole flight.

We checked into the hotel room, and a shuttle took us to the hospital, where I met Dr. Smith. He ran the tilt table test, and I passed out immediately. He then checked me into the hospital, and I was put on two different drugs. After three days he ran the tilt table test again. This time he put all kinds of different drugs in me through an IV, but I still passed out. He confirmed I had a bad case of neurocardiogenic syncope. He said I was in the top 2 percent of the severity of the condition. He then sent me back to the hotel on two other medications. I had a reaction to the medications. I thought I would go out of my mind. I was walking up and down the halls in my gown. I ended up in the emergency room on IVs, oxygen, and monitors. That was a really bad day for Ken and me, especially since we were so far from home.

When I think back, I find myself laughing about the memory of the tilt table test. I was put into this room and told to take off all my clothes and cover up with a sheet. They moved me from the bed to a stretcher so they could wheel me into the procedure room. As I was wheeled in, I immediately noticed all the monitors, X-ray machines, and what looked like a very thin table. A young man entered the room and said, "I need to get you ready for the test." He began to place electrical patches all over my back, neck, arms, ankles, legs, and chest—probably around forty patches. So there I was, completely nude on a cold, hard table with wires and patches all over me. I just wanted to be covered up. The doctor cut an incision in my groin and ran a wire through my body into my heart to measure my heart rate and blood pressure.

There I was, nude and Velcroed to a table with a very young guy and several lady nurses around me. Then the nurse picked up the phone, and I heard him say, "She's ready." Lo and behold, more people came walking in with notepads and pens with the doctor. Great day.

I was now completely nude, Velcroed to a table like a fly to a sticky strip, and the subject of observation for more than twenty people. A nurse said, "During the procedure, we play music. What kind do you like?"

I said, "Christian or gospel."

He said, "Either country or rock."

So I said, "Country."

Great. Now I was nude, Velcroed to a table, the subject of observation for twenty people, and listening to country music.

The nurse said, "Relax." *Yeah, right.*

All of a sudden, the table I was on started to tilt upward. I felt like I was in a space shuttle. All the monitors were beeping and humming; then I passed out. Remember, all of this was being done with country music in the background—"Yippy, Yiah!"

Days later, Ken and I headed for home. I was very upset. After all, I was going home with the right diagnosis but no treatment to help me. We were both upset. I had to go home, and nothing had changed.

As I entered the house, my children were there to see me. It hurt to see those sweet little faces welcoming me home. I'd had hopes of coming home with a cure, or at least a way to control my condition, but I had neither. I drew from God's Word: "Be strong and take heart, all you who hope in the Lord" (Psalm 31:24, NIV).

Shortly after coming home, I was so sick that it had gotten too hard to take the kids to our usual church. There was a church we could see from our front door: Pepperell Baptist Church. So we joined there. I remember the kids walking over there while

I crawled to the door and watched them go inside. I wanted so much to attend church, but I didn't want to pass out. There were many times I tried and started to get ready, but I would pass out before I finished getting dressed. I longed to go to church and would sit on the floor in front of the window and look at the steeple.

Saturdays and Sundays were the only days I had to rest before returning to work on Mondays. By Friday, I was always totally exhausted and just plain sick. For the next year I continued to struggle to work and take care of my family; it seemed impossible. I prayed, "Lord send me a local doctor who can help me."

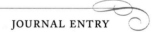

JOURNAL ENTRY

Dear Lord,

Thank you for helping me find a doctor who specializes in dysauotnomia. Even though my tests came out very bad, I trust in you, Lord, to help me through this. I want to be well for myself and my family. It breaks my heart every time I pass out and open my eyes and see two sweet faces looking at me with scared eyes. Give Tricia and Kenneth and Ken the strength they need to get through these difficult days. I am strong because I have you to lean on. Thank you, Lord. I love you, Lord.

Lynn

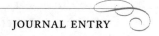

JOURNAL ENTRY

Dear Lord,

I am so afraid of having to live with this condition. Help me to be able to work and take care of my family. Give me your strength because I am afraid and have no strength. I love you.

Lynn

One Hot Summer Day

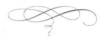

In 1 Timothy, chapter 4, the scripture from Paul to Timothy offers hope and comfort to keep Timothy on the right path. Verse 7 says, "Train yourself to be godly." It wasn't until I lost my physical abilities that I learned how valuable it was to be godly. Being sick forced me to focus on God and being godly instead of focusing on my physical self.

I continued to try to work and take care of my family and myself. But on one hot summer day in August 1994, I worked all day then went to teach Vacation Bible School that night. In one brief moment, I collapsed. I couldn't sit up. It felt like the blood was rushing out of my head. I felt weak, dizzy, and sick. I couldn't even sit up long enough to go home.

For hours, the preschool director, the pastor, and other church members sat around hoping and praying that soon I would be able to sit up and remain conscious. Since I lived only a block from the church, they ended up pushing me in a wheelchair while they leaned it back. I will never forget the terrified look on my son's face. He was only six years old at the time and was very frightened, as we all were. That was the last day I lived a normal life, the last day I worked or drove a car. All of a sudden, I could not do anything.

Before that my days had been spent waking up, getting out of bed, taking a shower, putting on makeup, fixing my hair, ironing clothes, keeping my house clean, and taking care of my children and husband. I admit that I was more concerned about my appearance than I was about my spiritual life. Yes, I attended church and loved my husband and kids, but on that hot summer day in August, my physical abilities died; only then did my spiritual abilities begin to blossom.

For the next several years, I lay in my bed, unable to get up without passing out. Over the next three years, I learned what it was to be godly. After all, whom could I lean on except God? I had lost my job, our savings, and my ability to go anywhere or take care of myself or my family. This forced me to spend more time with God praying and reading his Word.

"Train yourself to be godly." Before, I thought I had it all: a good job, a hard-working husband, two sweet children, a church, and a savings account. You might think that life sounded great, but without a personal relationship with God, you can't be godly or teach your children how to be godly.

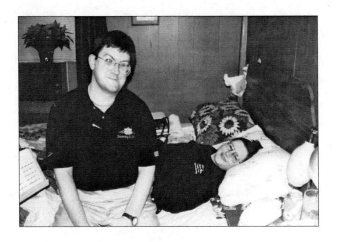

My life before had been a physical one, not a spiritual one. Look at verse 8 from the same chapter of 1 Timothy: "For physical training is of some value." *Some* value—that means little value. Verse 8 continues, "But godliness has value for all things." Wow! *All* things, not some things. So why had I spent more time on how I looked on the outside than on being godly? Perhaps it is the world we live in.

Listen. No matter how good you look, it can never replace the joy of a godly life. The rest of verse 8 goes on to say, "But godliness has value for all things, holding promise for both the present life and the life to come." What else has value for this life *and* the eternal life? Nothing! You can't take your looks or your money with you to heaven. Verses 9 and 10 say, "This is a trustworthy saying that deserves full acceptance. And for this we labor and strive that we have put our hope in the living God, who is the Savior of all men, and especially of those who believe." I have truly learned to put my hope in God. I experienced firsthand what it was like not to have anything to hope in but God.

You are probably wondering how I could stay completely in bed for years and not go crazy. How could I not be able to stand up next to my children and see how they had grown? How did I lie there day after day, year after year? It was because of my hope in God. I believe in him. Even though I had not given him much of my time previously, he still forgave me for my sins. He still loved me. When others gave up, God never did. Like Paul tells Timothy in verse 6, "Point these things out to your brothers."

Life as I knew it had ended. Unable to sit, stand, or work, suddenly I wanted to feel the breeze on my face and see the birds in the sky, but I was bedridden. I just wanted to be a good mother and wife and teach at church. I wanted to be in the world, but suddenly I was taken out of the world and forced to be bedridden and trapped in my own room.

> Do not love the world or anything in the world. If anyone loves the world, the love of the Father is not in him. For everything in the world the cravings of sinful man the lust of his eyes and the boasting of what he has and does comes not from the Father but from the world. The world and its desires pass away but the man who does the will of God lives forever.
>
> 1 John 2:15–17, NIV

Amen. That verse is so true. Things of the world can bring happiness for only a little while. Evil things also come from the world and are of the world. Through God, good things happen, and he never changes like the world does. Thank goodness for that. Could you imagine Jesus not being the same? What if he changed with the world? We would all be in trouble. That hot summer day, I truly learned what it was like to be godly.

JOURNAL ENTRY

Dear Lord,

This has been the most horrible day of my life. I collapsed, and I do not know what to do. I just want to sit up but can't without passing out. Lord, help me. My husband and children are frightened. This is so hard; I can't get up to help my family at all. I can't fix their lunches for school or wash their clothes or cook. Lord, what will become of us? Help us, Lord.

I love you.
Lynn

Second Trip to See Dr. Smith

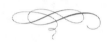

The second time I needed to go see Dr. Smith was a time when miracles happened—answered prayers. When I say *answered,* I mean quickly and exactly. At the time there was only a handful of doctors in the USA who treated people with dysautonomia. Dr. Smith was one of the leading doctors. Since my health had changed drastically, he wanted to see me again. My collapse the previous year and bedridden status since then would make it harder to travel. Over the previous year, Dr. Smith had been treating me over the phone, which had also been very difficult.

Ken and I began to pray for God's guidance. One problem was that it would cost around $2,200 to fly and for Ken to stay. We continued to pray and wait for God's answer. We used to leave our front door unlocked because at the time we lived across the street from our church and people came to check on me. This particular week, our next-door neighbors were having some trouble with the law, so Ken had locked the doors.

That morning, I did my usual Bible reading and devotion. I can remember what the scripture verse was "Greater love has no one than this, that he lay down his life for his friends" (John 15:13, NIV). I prayed again whether to go and see Dr. Smith. I began to feel bad, so I took a long nap. I woke as Ken entered for lunch. I picked up my Bible and began to read a little more. As I opened to the same scripture, I saw six one-hundred-dollar bills. I thought, *Wow. Lord, I know you want me to go see Dr. Smith.* Still, we needed eighteen hundred more dollars to make the trip. I said, "Ken, hurry. Come in here. Look. Did you put this money in my Bible?"

He said no and left.

I said, "Where are you going?"

He said, "To look in my Bible!"

Still, to this day, we do not know how the money appeared in my Bible. As for the rest of the money, Pepperell Baptist Church took up a love offering, which just happened to amount to eighteen hundred dollars.

God does answer prayers if you believe—truly believe—and love him with all your heart, soul, and mind. "Jesus replied: 'Love the Lord your God with all your heart and with all your soul and with your entire mind'" (Matthew 22:37, NIV).

Ken and I flew out to see Dr. Smith again. I had to lean on Ken the whole flight so I wouldn't pass out. Dr. Smith had an ambulance waiting to pick us up at the airport. I barely made it. It was good to lie down.

There I was again, getting my hopes up that there would be a cure or some medicine to help. It was snowing there and cold, so I did better on the tilt table test than the previous year. Having IV fluids the night before also helped my blood pressure. I wanted to believe that God had healed me. I could feel his presence with me throughout the test. However, the doctor said that the cold weather helped. Since I was given IV fluids, I felt that the test was not accurate because I couldn't receive them at home.

Even though I did better that visit, I still passed out with a very low blood pressure reading. Dr. Smith decided to try physical therapy, but I kept passing out. There was nothing else he could do for me, so I would continue to pray for a local cardiologist to help me instead of one that lived so far away. "Be joyful in hope, patient in affliction, faithful in prayer" (Romans 12:12, NIV).

While I was there, I witnessed to his nurse, Kerri. She asked me, "How do you stay so positive through all this?" I told her about God and how he could comfort her in any trouble she might have, like he had comforted me. She said she had never seen anything like it. I told her that with God anything is possible, even being positive in the midst of illness. The hospital also had cameras in every room, so when I prayed she saw it on the monitors and asked me about prayer.

After two weeks of physical therapy, Ken and I flew home. I still communicated with Kerri over the phone and continued to tell her about Jesus. It was difficult because I had to start from the beginning. She knew nothing of Jesus. I felt strongly about continuing to witness to Kerri.

Meanwhile, my heart started to race and beat very fast almost daily. Dr. Smith was worried about my mitral valve prolapse and the hole in my heart. He arranged for me to go to my local hospital and have an echocardiogram. They recorded my echocardiogram and sent it to Dr. Smith.

I was still witnessing to Kerri. Well, I had a thought. I would videotape myself and speak about Jesus, from his birth to dying for our sins then rising from the dead. This was all God's plan. The only problem was that I needed someone to tape me, and I did not own a camcorder. Ken happened to have some extra blank VHS tapes at our house. Then a friend, Cora, stopped by to check on me, and she happened to have a VHS camcorder in her car. It was God at work. She went outside and got it and taped me talking about Jesus and how to be saved. I quoted and referenced Scripture all throughout the video, and I also prayed a prayer for her to accept Jesus Christ as her savior. I couldn't wait to send it.

Another friend, Brenda, stopped by, and I asked her to mail Kerri the tape. The only address I had was Dr. Smith's office, so she mailed it there. I kept anticipating her call. I kept praying I could help her know about Jesus and how to become saved. "For

God so loved the world that he gave his one and only son, that whoever believes in him will not perish but have eternal life" (John 3:16, NIV).

A week went by, and she finally called. She said, "Lynn, you will never guess what happened." She stated how the doctor had received the video of my echo, and how he had sat down with his student residents to look at it. Only, to their surprise, it wasn't the echo. It was me telling Kerri how to be saved. She said, "One of the residents got up to turn the video off, and Dr. Smith said no." They all had to sit there and listen to me talking about Jesus Christ. Kerri received the echo video instead of the video I made for her about Jesus.

After that, Dr. Smith called not only to check on me but also to talk about God and eventually about how to be saved. I purchased him a Bible and mailed it. One day he called while Brenda was visiting me. After talking to him again about Jesus, he asked Jesus Christ into his heart while he and I were on the phone. Brenda and I were crying with joy. We finally knew the reason I had found Dr. Smith in the first place.

You see, God always has a plan. Even through trials, he can use you to teach others about Jesus. It was truly a miracle. Although I was still sick and bedridden, I felt joy knowing that God was using me for his glory. "'For I know the plans I have for you,' declares the Lord, 'plans to prosper you and not to harm you, plans to give you hope and a future'" (Jeremiah 29:11, NIV).

It was truly a miracle. This experience gave me a lot of hope because I knew God had plans for my life. Whom would you want to plan your life—yourself, your husband, your relatives, or God? As for me, I want God to plan my life. His plans will give me hope, and they will help me prosper. "Jesus looked at them and said, 'With man this is impossible, but with God all things are possible'" (Matthew 19:26, NIV).

"Jesus replied, 'What is impossible with men is possible with God'" (Luke 18:27, NIV).

Isn't that great? If we only had man to rely on, we wouldn't get very far. We as humans fade away. We sin and change with the world. But with God, anything is possible. God's plan might not be my plan, but I know that what he has in store for me is for my good.

My doctor asked Jesus Christ into his heart.

"The Lord gives strength to the weary and increases the power of the weak" (Isaiah 40:29, NIV). There I was, totally weak, and God made me strong. His grace and power helped me witness to my doctor. The Lord gave me the strength I didn't have.

JOURNAL ENTRY

Dear Lord,

Thank you for the opportunity to see Dr. Smith again. I am afraid because I am still sick. Physical therapy is only working a little. I want to be able to work, sit up, and get on with my life. Give my husband and children the strength they need to get through this. They have lost the mom they knew as active. I won't give up, Lord, because I know you have a mighty plan that I cannot see at this time. I love you, Lord. Thank you for saving Dr. Smith. If that is the reason I am ill, then it is okay, because he will go to heaven now when he dies. You are awesome, oh Lord.

The Trial Drug

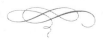

In 1995 Dr. Little moved from Birmingham to Florence, Alabama. Florence was a five-hour drive away. Ken and I tried to travel to see him every three months, but the five-hour drive each way was too much for me to handle. So Dr. Little found me a cardiologist in Montgomery: Dr. Crawford. She seemed knowledgeable about dysautonomia, but she was still an hour away. An hour-long ride in a bumpy ambulance was torture, but I took several ambulance rides to see her.

One time a friend, Heather, went with me in the ambulance. I passed out, and the paramedics couldn't detect a blood pressure. They were not sure what to do, so Heather told them to put ice all over me. Fortunately, it raised my blood pressure.

Meanwhile, as I got worse, Dr. Smith heard about a study at the University of Alabama at Birmingham for people with dysautonomia, but you had to have the condition severely. The study involved a drug called Proamatine. Dr. Smith called the doctor, and I qualified.

So we went to see yet another doctor: Dr. Cecil Coughlin. After running his own tests, he agreed with my other doctors. All of them said I had dysautonomia in the form of neurocardiogenic syncope. I prayed that this doctor would be able to help me. I prayed that the new study drug would help me be able to work and take care of my family. Dr. Coughlin was amazing and up in years. He had donated his whole life to treating and studying dysautonomia.

He told me I could be in the study. I would have to travel to Birmingham once a month to get the drug and be monitored; then I would return home. One rainy day, Brenda took me to Birmingham for the study drug, and I ended up passing out while she was driving on a two-lane highway in the rain. The problem was that I just tumbled into her lap. She had to pull the car over and move me off of her and try to get me conscious. I am happy to say we finally did make it home safely.

The drug gave me hope and helped me stand up without fainting or feeling like I was going to faint. It only lasted awhile, though. My doctor said my body had gotten used to the drug, and he was not comfortable increasing the dosage, for fear of overdosing. I told the Lord that all I wanted to do was walk, work, not be dizzy, not black out, and be normal.

Another day, my son wanted to play Cowboys

and Indians with me, so he shot me with a toy gun. I passed out, and he thought he had killed me. What a scared little boy!

I continued to get sicker and sicker. All I could do was pray and lean on God. I had seen enough doctors and definitely had a diagnosis, but I needed a doctor who was willing to do research, one who would be willing to try new things to help me and other sufferers. I have always felt that God wanted me to be a voice for the one million Americans who suffer from different types of dysautonomia.

"God is our refuge and strength, an ever-present help in trouble" (Psalm 46:1, NIV).

"The Lord is my strength and my shield; my heart trusts in him, and I am helped" (Psalm 28:7, NIV).

Strength, trust, and rest—I needed them all. I was losing control over my body but not my spirit. I wanted to see Dr. Coughlin regularly, but he already had so many patients from all over the United States that he couldn't fit me in. I prayed every night for a doctor who would help people with dysautonomia in Alabama, Georgia, and the surrounding states.

"Jesus said, 'My grace is sufficient for you, for my power is made perfect in weakness'" (2 Corinthians 12:9, NIV). God's grace was sufficient for me. What else would be? When I was physically weak, I became spiritually powerful. It felt so good to have God to lean on while trying a new drug. He guided me through it all.

"My soul finds rest in God alone; my salvation comes from him" (Psalm 62:1, NIV). We cannot get our salvation from anyone else. We should just rest and not worry. Find rest in God and God alone.

Even though I kept getting sicker and sicker, God still had a plan for my life. It wasn't my choice but his. Being able to participate in the trial was a blessing. It helped me feel better for a little while, and I thanked God for those times.

I continued to remain bedridden. I stayed in my dark room day after day, month after month, year after year from 1994 until 1998. I was too sick to travel to see the cardiologist in Montgomery, and the ambulance drive was not covered by insurance. So I lay in the bed. What else could I do? Every time I got up, I passed out, sometimes hurting myself. People from Pepperell Baptist Church came over and checked on me. Often, my friends found me passed out on the floor. I couldn't give up. I wanted to walk.

The next several years would be very difficult. I was getting worse. I had lost my job and my abilities to care for my husband and children. That broke my heart because I loved my family so much. I just wanted to be a good wife and a good mother. All I ever wanted for my life was to raise godly children and share Jesus with others.

One day my parents came from Florida for a visit. It was always hard on me when they came because they didn't accept that I was sick. This visit was extra hard because I wanted so much to please them and be well, but I couldn't. No matter how hard I tried, I was just simply sick. So there I was in my room, unable to get up without passing out, and my mother and father came to visit. My mother said, "Lynn, get out of that bed. This is so silly." Ken tried to explain my condition and why I wasn't out of bed, as he had done so many times before, but my parents wouldn't accept that or me.

They came to my room. I crawled off the bed and onto my knees, trying not to pass out. I said, "Mom and Dad, I love you both. Please accept me the way I am. I didn't choose to be sick and stuck in bed. I can't help it." They both said that they couldn't and wouldn't accept me, so what was I to do? Would I let them continue to hurt me verbally? My parents got angry that I wouldn't get out of bed, so they left, leaving behind two very upset grandchildren.

Over the years, I kept trying to get them to understand my condition and accept me. It was hard not having support from my parents, but it only got worse. My mother returned to my hometown, where she lived. She told people I was just weak from lying in bed, that I wasn't actually sick. This resulted in the loss of so many of my friends and family members. It hurt so badly that people were dropping out of my life like flies, people whom I had loved and spent time with my whole life. I never heard from my aunts, uncles, cousins on my mom's side of the family, or my brother. Soon, not only my family ignored me, but my hometown friends started to tell me to get up, having the same attitude my mom had. This would be something I struggled with for years.

I tried everything. I printed information on the condition. I talked and talked, but nothing worked. I needed to give it to the Lord. My problem was that I didn't leave it in the Lord's hands. I kept picking it back up. After all, I wanted my children to have grandparents, but I couldn't pretend I was well like my parents wanted. Many times when they visited I took extra medication so I could sit up while they were there. I was risking my life, and for what—a smile, a nod of approval from my mom? I couldn't keep trying to be someone else just to please them. I had to stop.

If you suffer from dysautonomia or a chronic illness, don't pretend you are well. Just be yourself, whether sick or well. I know that is hard to do because I have been there. Just always tell the truth. You cannot control what someone else thinks. All that matters is what God thinks. I was *Lynn*. God had made me different for a reason, and he loved and accepted me just the way I was.

"Let the beloved of the Lord rest secure in him, for he shields him all day long, and the one the Lord loves rests between his shoulders" (Deuteronomy 33:12, NIV).

"Nothing will be able to separate us from the love of God that is in Christ Jesus our Lord" (Romans 8:38, NIV).

I am so glad the Lord loves me and lets me rest in him all day long. Wow! Romans 8:39 says, neither height nor depth, nor anything else in all creation, will be able to separate us from the love of God that is in Christ Jesus our Lord. Nothing can separate us from the love of God. If you have lost family too, remember this scripture.

Also read Psalm 136. See how many times the Bible says his love endures forever. God loves us so much that he sent his son into the world to save us from our sins. That is how I know God loves me, and he loves you too. His love endures forever.

JOURNAL ENTRY

Dear Lord,

Even though my parents do not accept me, I still love them. I am asking you to help them understand and accept my condition. I certainly do not want to feel this way. I feel so sick every day. It gets harder and harder. I know what your Bible says, that no one can separate me from your love. I am thankful for that. Shower me with your love as I grieve for my family to love and accept me. I am thankful for Ken, Tricia, and Kenneth, who love me no matter what. I know this isn't easy on them. Help them, Lord. Thank you, Lord, for Dr. Cecil Coughlin, who is willing for me to take the experimental drug Proamatine. I greatly admire all the work he has done over the years helping people who suffer. He is amazing. Give us all strength. Help this drug to help other sufferers of dysautonomia. Thank you for everything you have given to me, Lord. I love you.

Declared Disabled

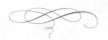

For six years, I had battled a medical condition and was trying to get on Social Security to offset my medical expenses and lost income. One day in October of 1996, my pastor and the youth minister decided to go to the Social Security office and fuss because it had been so long and there I was, unable to get up and having seizures. My pastor at the time spoke harshly to the lady, and the youth minister had to remind him he was a pastor. But the lady told him I had gotten on Social Security. So they finally declared me disabled, backing it up to the year 1995. The doctors told me there was no other drug to try, and they had done all they could do for me. I felt my whole life ending.

Do you know what being officially, legally *disabled* means? It means to take away your physical abilities. My freedom to be able to work or to drive had ended. My independence and physical life had changed. Just going to the store was a challenge.

However, this did not mean I was disabled spiritually. Actually, I was growing closer to the Lord. I had been spending so much time with God that I could feel his presence more than ever before. My prayer life grew 100 percent.

We had a canopy bed, and all underneath the canopy I taped Scripture so I could see them while lying down. I read them all several times each day:

> May your unfailing love be my comfort, according to your promise to your servant.
>
> Psalm 119:76, NIV

> The Lord is my rock my fortress and my deliverer; my God is my rock, in whom I take refuge. He is my shield and the horn of my salvation, my stronghold.
>
> Psalm 18:2, NIV

> I love you, O Lord, my strength.
>
> Psalm 18:1, NIV

> A horse is a vain hope for deliverance; despite all its great strength it cannot save. But the eyes of the Lord are on those whose hope is in his unfailing love, to deliver them from death and keep them alive in famine.
>
> Psalm 33:17–19, NIV

I am not afraid to die physically because I will not die spiritually. I can't wait to see Jesus. God gave his only Son to die and suffer for our sins so that, through him, we will be saved.

My son had been to the revival at our church. He came home and ran into my bedroom and held out his sweet little hand. He was around seven years old at the time. He was very upset and crying. I asked him, "What's wrong?"

He held out his hand and said, "Mommy, don't you know that it had to hurt Jesus when they put that nail through his hand." He was so sweet with tears coming out of his big, brown eyes. Childlike faith—it was wonderful. If Jesus can suffer the way he did, I can certainly endure some pain. I believe some people suffer as a sacrifice to show others their love for God. They can either be bitter about being sick or better—spiritually better.

> So do not be ashamed to testify about our Lord, or ashamed of me his prisoner. But join with me in suffering for the gospel, by the power of God. Who has saved us and called us to a holy life, not because of anything we have done but because of his own purpose and grace. This grace was given us in Christ Jesus before the beginning of time.
>
> 2 Timothy 1:8–9, NIV

> It is granted to you on behalf of Christ not only to believe on him, but also to suffer for him, since you are going through the same struggle you saw I had, and now hear that I still have.
>
> Philippians 1:29–30, NIV

It is better, if it is God's will to suffer for doing good than for doing evil. For Christ died for sins once for all, the righteous for the unrighteous to bring you to God. He was put to death in the body but made alive by the Spirit, though whom also he went and preached to the spirits in prison.

1 Peter 3:17–19, NIV

You could say my physical body was put to death. At least, it didn't work anymore, but my spiritual life thrived. I have always tried to do well but just did not spend enough time with God. All of a sudden, my spirit was coming alive while my physical body was fading away.

"Dear friends, do not be surprised at the painful trial you are suffering, as though something strange were happening to you. But rejoice that you participate in the sufferings of Christ, so that you may be overjoyed when his glory is revealed" (1 Peter 4:12–13, NIV). This Bible verse is so true; I thought something strange was happening to me. The Bible tells us not to be surprised at painful trials. Just trust in God and lean on him, not your understanding. After all, you are doing something Jesus Christ did, and that is suffering. You have something in common with Jesus. Who else would you rather have something in common with?

"Trust in the Lord with all your heart and lean not on your own understanding; in all your ways acknowledge him. And he will make your paths straight" (Proverbs 3:5–6, NIV).

Sometimes we just think too much. We try to

have an answer for every little thing when we should trust in the Lord with everything. It doesn't matter if we understand. I didn't understand why I was so sick, but God was making my path straight where he wanted it. I just had to trust in him. That certainly didn't mean it was easy. But if God is your strength, you can live above your illness.

"Look to the Lord and his Strength; seek his face always" (1 Chronicles 16:11, NIV).

JOURNAL ENTRY

Dear Lord,

Becoming disabled is such a bad feeling. It is when you certainly have to admit you are too ill to work. I loved my job. But I couldn't keep passing out at work, and now that I am bedridden, I certainly cannot work. Lord, I pray to you to find me the right doctor. I am leaning on your strength for that. I trust in you and your love for me. I am going through a terrible trial right now, and I know in time your glory will be revealed. Especially help and bless my children and husband with your love. I love you, Lord. Please help me.

You Are Not Crazy

Some people who have dysautonomia are told they need psychiatric help. When their doctors cannot explain their physical condition, the first alternative is, "It's in your head." What is the definition of *crazy* anyway? Your mind and body both go together. When physically, you cannot control your blood pressure, then you cannot think straight. Most of the time you only have five minutes or so to talk with your busy doctor. That isn't enough time to determine your condition physically or mentally.

Be sure your doctor takes time to hear you. While many symptoms of dysautonomia do mimic depression, don't let it make you doubt yourself. Think back to before you started passing out. Did you fight depression then? Examine yourself. If you are depressed, seek help, but if you know something physically is not right, say it. It has been my experience that most people with dysautonomia were happy and active until the condition crept into their lives. When a physical condition such as dysautonomia controls your life, yes, you can *become* depressed. However, it is second to your physical condition. Don't let a doctor, family member, or friend tell you that you are emotionally or mentally ill unless it is true. Have control over yourself; examine yourself physically, spiritually, and emotionally.

As for myself, I had several different opinions. In the 1990s the condition was hardly known by any physicians. I had been bedridden for two years and was getting worse. In 1996 I got so bad I couldn't stop having seizures. I was taken to East Alabama Medical Center and put in the intensive care unit. I was so sick I had to ride in an ambulance to Montgomery to see a neurologist. He said, "You are sick from lying in bed." He didn't know any better because he was not trained on the condition of dysautonomia.

I had become so weak I was passing out. How did he think I ended up in bed in the first place? I felt like he was crazy along with everyone else. I would pass out just by sitting up. It was horrible! I let the neurologist and my family convince me I was just weak. My parents took what he said like water to a sponge. I knew I was sick, but they listened to an untrained doctor instead.

I am sure it is hard for a family member to watch a loved one suffer from a rare, as yet undiagnosed condition. But seeing a neurologist for dysautonomia back then was like going to see a dentist because you are pregnant. Over the last decade, more and more neurologists and cardiologists have come to learn more about dysautonomia. That is something I had prayed for all along. I should have spoken up and left the hospital. What they actually did was get my hopes up. The neurologist, along with Dr. Crawford, decided to send me to a rehabilitation hospital.

I was taken off all medications and forced to sit up. I was treated like a child. I was told, "Don't lie down. Get up." I felt so bad, but I thought, *maybe I'm just weak. Wouldn't that be great!* This gave me hope that I would walk again without fainting.

I was taken to the rehabilitation hospital by ambulance. As I entered, I only saw elderly people. It seemed more like a nursing home. A rehabilitation doctor came in my room and said, "There's no reason why you can't be up." I didn't say a word, but I should have.

A physical therapist came in and started working with me on lifting my head and sitting upright. Of course, I was weak, but that wasn't what caused me to stay in bed in the first place. It was a very, very low blood pressure that kept me bedridden. My organs couldn't get the proper blood flow. I was given a wheelchair and preached to: "Don't lie in bed. Go to therapy, and wheel yourself." Boy was that hall long; it was bad to see ninety- and eighty-year-old people doing better than I was, and I was in my thirties. I got in the wheelchair, and slowly I went up and down the halls. I felt so bad I cried the whole time. Everything would go black. It was awful.

My physical therapist worked hard with me. I started passing out when I tried to walk. Why must I argue and convince them I had a physical condition? I felt it; I knew my blood pressure was not stable. One minute I was getting fussed at; the next I was told not to get out of bed. My therapist decided to put a heart monitor on me with a blood pressure cuff. After she saw what happened when I stood, she started recording it. I was told I'd be at the rehabilitation hospital for nine weeks. After they saw what my body did when upright, they said, "We have done all we can do for you." But they had already convinced my family I wasn't sick.

If you have been told it is all in your head, I understand what you are going through. It just plain hurts when you are not heard. Don't let anyone tell you that you are crazy. You know your own heart, mind, and soul. I thank the Lord I had him to lean on. I took the opportunity to witness while I was there. God had me there to motivate others. I had a devotional book with me and spent time going from room to room. I kept passing out, but I never gave up on sharing Jesus Christ with others.

I remember once while in a support group one elderly lady was crying because she had to leave her little dog behind when she came to the rehabilitation hospital. The therapist had lost control of the session. I spoke up to her. "You are my hero. I remember the first day I came here; you could wheel down the hall with the use of only one leg and one arm. You inspired me." She just needed Jesus' love. When I left the session, the doctor stopped me and thanked me for helping to calm the woman down.

When I first arrived, I didn't want Ken to leave me there. I stayed in my room and ate. I prayed to God to help me. After I prayed, I gathered the strength to go into my area to eat with the others. At first, the elderly wouldn't have anything to do with me. I would smile and sit at a table with them, but they would get up and leave me sitting alone. I felt like I didn't fit in there. I knew God loved me; I always fit in his hands. It wasn't long before the elderly patients were fighting to sit at my table. I couldn't eat myself for having to open ketchup, butter, and sugar packets for everyone else. Everyone started to find out it was good to have a young person around to help them.

There was one special man there named James. He had previously had a stroke and couldn't talk or use his hands or walk. I noticed as I wheeled past him that his eyes would watch me. I started talking to him, helping him eat, and praying with him. Several weeks later, I wheeled by his room. I had passed out and was very weak, but I was still trying. As I wheeled by his room, he lifted up his hand for me. He was crying and all alone. An aide told me that his wife had just died, and he could not go to her funeral.

There he was, trapped in a body that couldn't speak or work right. He was taken away from his home, and his wife had just died, but he couldn't go to the funeral. His eyes met mine, and although he couldn't talk, I knew how he was feeling. I wheeled into his room. I wasn't strong enough to hold up my head. I laid my head on his bed and held his hand. He cried, and I cried. Even though we couldn't carry on a conversation, I felt his spirit. We connected. I stayed with him for over an hour. I asked him, "Did your wife know Jesus?" His eyes brightened. I told him she was okay. She was in heaven. He tried to smile out of his paralyzed face. Even though we hadn't known each other long, it was one of the most meaningful times I had ever had spiritually. There we were, being still with God.

I also went to a Sunday worship service at the rehabilitation hospital. It had been so long since I had attended church. This was something I had prayed for. I wheeled into the room and noticed a nice, clean-cut gentleman, who was the preacher. I also saw a man playing soul music on the piano. We shouted to the Lord. It was one of the most meaningful church services I had ever attended. I was praising God and holding hands with two complete strangers, but I could feel God in their hearts. Some had no legs, or arms, or droopy faces due to strokes. "The Lord is my Shepherd." That is what we all shouted, and it was glorious. I wept with joy. I learned that a big, pretty church didn't matter; that a church service was made up of the people worshiping God and praising his name. It was amazing how the Spirit was in the room.

I had two different roommates, and both enriched my life in many ways. We laughed together and cried together. The day Ken came to take me home, there was a whole hall of people crying. We had become like family. Ken said, "I hate to take you home. Everyone is upset and crying. They all need you."

I hadn't reached my goal. I could only take a few steps on the parallel bars. I wasn't walking, but I had shared Jesus with many people. It didn't matter who said it was all in my head. I knew the truth, and the truth finally came out. They never actually said I was crazy, but I knew they thought I was nuts if I wanted to lie flat all day and night.

"To the Jews who had believed him, Jesus said, 'if you hold to my teaching, you are really my disciples. Then you will know the truth, and the truth will set you free'" (John 8:31–32, NIV).

After leaving the hospital, I was sent back to see Dr. Crawford. She put me back on all my medication and said she was sorry for sending me there, that there just wasn't enough information on the condition to know not to try the rehabilitation hospital. Even though the doctor said I wasn't sick they put me in a rehabilitation hospital, and the truth ended up setting me free. When I kept passing out, everyone saw the truth, and that put everything back in order. No more false hope. I know myself and my body more than anyone other than God.

Doctors are only human. We forget that at times. Working together with your doctor is the best way to help yourself. Even though it was difficult being told I could walk when I couldn't, God had a plan to use me to witness to people at the rehabilitation hospital. That is why I am here on earth: to help others. I am here for God, to show people God loves them and they are special in his eyes. Witnessing to others was the thing that got me through such a difficult time in my life. But I still knew somewhere there was a doctor who could help me, who would at least listen to me and believe in me. I continued to pray for that daily.

JOURNAL ENTRY

Dear Lord,

It is so hard not to be heard. I knew I had a physical condition. But I was treated unjustly just because a doctor was not trained about my condition. I know there are many people who have been treated the same way. Staying at the rehabilitation hospital was like a nightmare. I felt so bad physically, but no one would listen until they put me on a heart monitor and saw for themselves what happened when I stood up. Lord, I know there are people with dysautonomia who are treated like the condition is all in their heads, but it's not. Help them find a doctor who is trained and can help them. No one would want to feel like I do. Thank you for the opportunity to help others and witness for you. When I witness, I feel I have a purpose in life, and that purpose is you. Thank you for helping me through such a difficult time in my life. Thank you for allowing me to help my friend when his sweet wife died.

Dad's Seventieth Birthday Party

For years I hadn't felt a part of my family's lives. When I say *family* I do not mean my husband and two children. They do love and accept me. But on this day I would find out I sure wasn't a part of my relatives' lives. It was March 22, 1997, my dad's seventieth birthday. It was supposed to be a day of joy, happiness, and laughter. We were celebrating seventy years of my dad's life.

Ken and I drove to Florida with our two children. The trip was so hard on me physically and emotionally; I had to lie down the whole way. I also cried the whole way there. I didn't want to go because my parents didn't accept my condition, but I did love and care about my dad. My aunt came from out of town and wanted to make it a huge event, the whole nine yards. My brother planned most of the party.

When I got out of the rehabilitation hospital in 1996, I was sent home with a wheelchair, and I tried to continue to use it. When we first arrived at my mom's house, she said, "You can't bring that wheelchair in my house. Leave it outside." I gathered then that she was embarrassed of me, and especially she didn't want her floor to have tire marks on it. She wanted everything to seem perfect. It might have been perfect for everyone else, but it wasn't for me.

I was told by my aunt, "Stand up and chop this. Cook that." I gathered she didn't understand what *disabled* meant. So I went into the restroom and took extra medication that would help me be able to stand briefly and sit up for longer periods of time. Once again, I risked my life to fit in.

The party was at a Baptist church. Ken and I drove there. As I entered I saw my aunts, uncles, and cousins, brother, sister-in-law, niece, and nephews, along with lifelong friends. I was ignored and looked at like I was crazy. You would have thought I had been in jail for killing someone.

My cousin walked over to me and said, "Get out of that wheelchair." That is what I wanted to do but couldn't, not for a long period of time. No one else spoke to me, even though it had been years since I had seen most of them. Only one aunt and one cousin spoke, and what each of them said were negative. I didn't feel a part of the family at all. I held back the tears and couldn't wait to get out of there.

I stayed in my wheelchair in the corner of the room. I had a lifelong friend say, "Don't sit in the wheelchair. You'll just get weaker." I wanted to burst into tears. I gathered they had been misinformed, but I would not start any conversation that might hurt my dad's party. What I should have done was leave. I should have gotten my children and my husband and left.

After the singing, eating, and socializing, my brother asked if anyone wanted to speak about my dad. I guess he had a reason to brag about his dad. Then my sister-in-law talked. My aunts also talked, along with friends and other relatives. I was the only person who didn't speak; I was holding back a flood of tears, so I said nothing. My brother and his wife didn't speak to me. Neither did my nephews or niece.

There was a lady there, though, who knew how I had been raised and knew the situation. Mrs. Duncan spoke up, saying, "Lynn is like one of my daughters, and I love her." It felt so good to hear that someone loved and accepted me. Mrs. Duncan was always there for me when I was growing up.

My cousin Sandy, my Uncle Hollis, and my Aunt Gloria came in late. I was relieved to see them. When I was little, my Aunt Gloria had always loved me, and my Uncle Hollis had always cared about me too. I thank the Lord for them.

As I am typing this, I still get tears in my eyes because I am disowned by my family over being sick. Everyone wanted to have their picture taken with my dad. I was told by my mom to get out of the wheelchair. Even though I felt so bad, I stood up long enough for a picture. My mother has this look on her face that sticks straight to my heart like a knife.

I have learned so much since that day in 1997. Today I wouldn't place myself in a position like that to be hurt. I don't waste my energy anymore trying to explain over and over what is wrong with my health. I have spent too many days being unaccepted. It has kept me from doing what God wanted me to do.

If you have a loved one or friend with dysautonomia, the best thing you can do for them is simply be there, love them, and accept them. If you have experienced what I have, then the Bible contains scripture that will help you.

> My heavenly Father, I desire to become mature, attaining to the whole measure of the fullness of Christ. For then I will no longer be an infant, tossed back and forth by the waves, and blown here and there by every wind of teaching and by the cunning and craftiness of men in their deceitful scheming. Instead, please teach me to speak the truth in love, growing up into Him who is the head that is Christ.
>
> Ephesians 4:13–15, NIV

You see, I should have spoken up. It wouldn't have mattered whether my family had believed I was ill. I would be speaking the truth. Not doing that, I let them believe the lies they were told. "Lord, your inspired word declares that the knowledge of your truth leads to godliness" (Titus 1:1, NIV).

"But you have planted wickedness, you have reaped evil, you have eaten the fruit of deception. Because you have depended on your own strength and on your many warriors" (Hosea 10:13, NIV). You diagnose the root of the problem by saying that they have eaten the fruit of deception. People like this depend on their own strength and on many other warriors. I asked God to help me not partake of the fruit of deception but to refuse it.

"In your majesty ride forth victoriously on behalf of truth, humility and righteousness; let your right hand display awesome deeds (Psalm 45:4, NIV).

David asks God to expose deeply to him the truth, to show him the lies he has believed and to help him replace them with *permanently* engraved truth. That is what we should do. Seek out the truth. Do not believe in lies. Go and see for yourself. Gossip and slander is like cancer; it grows and grows. So many lies were spread about me that my relatives did not accept me. "Lord, do not allow anything or anyone to snatch the word of truth from my mouth, oh Lord, for I have put my hope in your laws" (Psalm 119:43, NIV).

That March day I let my family snatch the truth away from me because I did not speak up like I should have. For my hope is in the truth and in God, not in my family. Study God's word on the truth. It will help you when someone doesn't accept you. Speak up and tell the truth. Do not sit silently like I did that horrible day. I think I must have cried for weeks after the party, but now I have a different perspective on the situation. God has helped me overcome the most hurtful day of my life.

If you are a relative or friend of a person who suffers from dysautonomia or some other chronic illness, here is a scripture that will help you.

> What good is it, brothers, if a man claims to have faith but has no deeds? Can such faith save him? Suppose a brother or sister is without clothes and daily food. If one of you says to him, "Go, I wish you well; keep warm and well fed," but does nothing about his physical needs, what good is it? In the same way, faith by itself, if it is not accompanied by action, is dead. But, someone will say, "You have faith; I have deeds." Show me your faith without deeds, and I will show you my faith by what I do. You believe that there is one God. Good! Even the demons believe that and shudder. You foolish man, do you want evidence that faith without deeds is useless? Was not our ancestor Abraham considered righteous for what he did when he offered his son Isaac on the Altar? You see that his faith and his actions were together, and his faith was made complete by what he did. And the scripture was fulfilled that says, "Abraham believed God, and it was credited to him as righteousness, and he was called God's friend." You see that a person is justified by what he does and not by faith alone. In the same way, was not even Rehab the prostitute considered righteous for what she did when she gave lodging to the spies and sent them off in a different direction?

As the body without the spirit is dead, so faith without deeds is dead.

James 2:14–26, NIV

You see, none of my relatives ever came to see me, to see for themselves how I was. They had no idea what my needs were. For over a decade, I never received a card, a phone call, or a visit. No action—the Bible says to have actions. My brother stopped by several times on his way home from vacation since he was driving through my town, but he never called even to ask how I was. I prayed for months and years for my aunts, uncles, parents, brother, and others to come see me, to believe in me.

If you have a loved one with dysautonomia, take action. Call. Send a card. Give money if needed. You could even help clean the house or the yard. It would mean the world to them because most of the people with dysautonomia just want to be accepted. You have the power to do that. Love them with the love God gives you. Faith without deeds is dead.

JOURNAL ENTRY

Dear Lord,

Today was one of the worst days of my life. My relatives didn't care about me. They didn't talk to me. I was treated so badly. I was just stared at and judged. I can only pray they will see the truth and love me no matter what. Everyone treated me like I was crazy, but I am not. I have tried time and time again to explain my condition, but each time, I have been ignored and not spoken to. It would have been wonderful if they had helped me through the last several years. But they did not. I know, Lord, that you believe in me and understand the pain I am going through, the pain of having my family not care. I am leaning on your love because you love me no matter if I am sick or well. Help and bless my husband and children. Thank you, God. You are awesome.

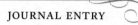

JOURNAL ENTRY

Dear Lord,

Even though I am disabled, my children can still learn to put you first in their lives. I pray my disability will not hurt them, but with your plan I hope it helps them be stronger by leaning on you. It is very hard to hear them struggling in the kitchen and all. I just want to jump up and help them cook. It is funny that even though I do not leave my bed, I can still tell them where things are when they can't find something. I guess I know how they think. I love you, Lord. Lynn

Friends

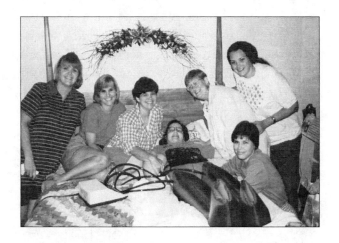

We all need friends. For several years I prayed for a friend, one who was also suffering with dysautonomia, not that I would wish this condition on anyone. But I reasoned that if I could find someone else who had it, I would know they understood what I was going through.

In October of 1997 a dear friend of mine bought me a computer. It would be my first computer, and it led me to my first friend with my condition. I told my friend I would use the computer he had given me for God's glory. And I kept to those words.

Every day I posted messages on the Internet. Every morning I signed on my computer and hoped I would hear from someone. I talked to my other friends about how I felt, but because they didn't suffer from the condition, they could not relate to me. One day I signed on the computer, and finally I had a message from "Becky." I sobbed as I read the e-mail from her. She said she was on the same medications I was on. She also said she was struggling to sit up without passing out, as I was. As I cried I had a feeling of relief. Someone understood. I knew from that day forward that I had to reach out to others with dysautonomia.

Through the years I have been a support leader, and I have made numerous books of hope for people with dysautonomia. I have had some friends on the Internet for ten years. Some have died, some have gotten better, and some remain the same.

All throughout the Bible, God talks about friends. Not only does he want us to have friends, but he also wants to be our friend. Over the years, I have e-mailed so many sufferers of dysautonomia. What is important is that, at least for a brief time, they felt comforted by my acceptance of them and the way I cared about them through Jesus's love.

"If you remain in me and my words remain in you …" (John 15:7, NIV).

I love and care about people who suffer from dysautonomia. But apart from God, nothing can be accomplished. So I must remain in God and show his love to others by caring about them and being their friend.

One day while I was looking on the Web site, I noticed an eighteen-year-old online. She sounded so desperate. She could not go to her high school or the prom or even drive. She seemed so lonely, saying she couldn't live on earth anymore. She wasn't making it. I e-mailed her, telling her that God loves her and that I cared about her and understood the struggles she was going through. The Bible says to comfort each other with the comfort we ourselves have felt. Just five minutes later, I received an e-mail from her. I was so glad to hear she was okay.

She said that she had a handful of pills and was ready to take them to end her life. She wrote, "You saved my life." She shared how she felt no one understood until I e-mailed her and shared that God loved her. She said her computer said, "You have mail," right before she put the pills in her mouth. She read my e-mail, which made her feel accepted and loved. What she needed was Jesus' love. Throughout the years, I have e-mailed and talked to her by phone, and I am very happy to say that she has been called by

God to be a missionary, and her health has improved. Glory to God!

God wants us to have friends. It says in the Bible to lay down your life for your friends (John 15:13, NIV).

"A friend loves at all times, and a brother is born for adversity" (Proverbs 17:17, NIV).

"A man of many companions may come to ruin, but there is a friend who sticks closer than a brother" (Proverbs 18:24, NIV).

I have had friends who have truly stuck by my side so much closer than my actual brother. My friends have loved me at all times, no matter if I am sick or well. Having Jesus in their hearts helps them to love in that way.

> Two are better than one, because they have a good return for their work: If one falls down, his friend can help him up. But pity the man who falls and has no one to help him up! Also, if two lie down together, they will keep warm. But how can one keep warm alone? Though one may be overpowered, two can defend themselves. A cord of three strands is not quickly broken.
>
> Ecclesiastes 4:9–12, NIV

Let's stick together. We need each other's warmth and compassion to help us through the terrible days. So many of my friends have gone through sad and happy times with me. Amen for that, because those of us with dysautonomia literally do fall down. I am thankful to my Lord for my friends. There have been so many times when friends have helped me.

One time I didn't answer the phone, and my friend Betty thought I was passed out. She rushed over with her hair in curlers and in her robe and was standing on the porch when my husband got home from buying groceries.

Another time I passed out, and it was so hot my blood pressure wouldn't rise, so my friend Judy put ice all over me, except the ice was in the form of frozen peas, corn, and other vegetables. When I came to, I said, "Are we having soup for lunch?"

Another time I woke up in a bathtub filled with ice to find several men looking at me. I am thankful they could come and put me in ice so my blood pressure would rise. That way I wouldn't suffer and stay passed out for as long. But being put in ice was always torture.

One time I passed out and my friend Tommye had to climb through a window to help me. Other times a friend would take me for a ride in his truck because I was going stir-crazy staying in the house so long, year after year. He and my husband would use a backboard to transport me. I can remember those rides through town, and if he got close to turning down my street, I would cry and beg him not to take me home. He would have the air conditioner so high there would be frost on it, and that was in the summer time. Another time I had been locked in my bedroom for two years. A dear friend, Mr. Furlow, put a bed in his motor home and took me to Callaway Gardens to see God's beauty. I will never forget what that meant to me. To have caring friends is a treasure from God.

One hot summer day, my electricity went off, and I began to get hot. With dysautonomia, you are not supposed to get hot. I called my friend Martha, and she came over in her robe, straight from her bed, and helped drag me into her van. She put the air conditioner in her van on high. It was a nightmare. I passed out on her. Bless her heart, she didn't give up, but helped me stay cool.

One summer day my friend couldn't find a blood pressure; I was passed out. So she called for some help to put me in the tub with cold water to raise my blood pressure. But the water wasn't running in the house, so they had to find a hose and hook it up to a neighbor's faucet and fill buckets of water until they had filled the tub. Then they put ice in. That is when my blood pressure rose, and I awoke to see around me five different people relieved I was finally conscious.

I have a friend named Patty, who takes me back and forth to doctor's appointments. One day when we arrived at my house, I passed out in her car. She had to find some men to carry my limp body into the house where I could be cooled off and hooked up to an IV so my blood pressure would rise.

Another day, my friend Judy was taking me to a doctor's appointment. She came in and got me in my wheelchair and pushed me outside the back door. My ramp is so steep and is straight down, kind of like a mini roller coaster. Well, I started to roll, and

I asked her if she had me. She turned around, and I was flying down the ramp. I was flying through the air. I put my hands out and ran right into her van, which was parked in the road. She had my handprints in the side of her van. I am thankful her van was there so that no one would run over me with a car. What a hoot!

It is a blessing to have friends who care about you and love you. God has truly blessed me with eternal friends.

> Carry each other's burdens, and in this way you will fulfill the law of Christ. If anyone thinks he is something when he is nothing, he deceives himself. Each one should test his own actions. Then he can take pride in himself, without comparing himself to somebody else, for each one should carry his own load.
>
> Galatians 6:2–5 (NIV)

It helps us when we carry each other's burdens because then we do not dwell on our own burdens. I thank God for all my friends who have carried my burdens all these years. When I say *years* I am talking about more than a decade that people have been helping me and my family.

"Let us not give up meeting together, as some are in the habit of doing, but let us encourage one another and all the more as you see the day approaching" (Hebrews 10:25, NIV). We need to encourage one another, especially the ones whom we have things in common with. That way, we can comfort them in the way we have been comforted by Jesus Christ.

Let God comfort you with his promises. You will feel better; maybe not well, but better. Having the support of friends is a gift from God. If you don't have many friends, pray for some. I did that at one time when I first moved to a new town. I prayed for friends, and now I have some. Christ changed us from enemies into his friends and gave us the task of making others his friends also. I know Christ wants to be your friend.

> You are my friends if you do what I command. I no longer call you servants, because a servant does not know his masters business. Instead, I have called you friends, for everything that I learned from my Father I have made known to you.
>
> John 15:14–15, NIV

You can count on God never leaving you and always accepting you.

JOURNAL ENTRY

Dear Lord,

Thank you so much for my friends who have come to my rescue when I was passed out and having seizures. Thank you for the ones who brought me lunch when I had none. Thank you for their loving me just the way I am. You have taught me that a friend can be closer than a brother. Friends are what have helped me through so many days of suffering. I am humbled, dear Lord.

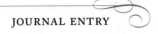

JOURNAL ENTRY

Lord,

Help people in the church to reach out to my children. I am thankful for every time Leigh has watched my kids while I was either in the hospital or sick. She helps me so much. Thank you, Lord, for Leigh. Thank you also for Earl and Wanda Barron, who have faithfully come over to help me. There are so many people at Pepperell who help Ken and me. I am glad Sue Peppers is in Tricia's life. She is like a grandmother to her.

A Letter to NASA
March 1997

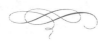

Dear Daniel S. Golden, Administrator of NASA:

I am a thirty-six-year-old wife and mother of two children. I suffer from a rare condition, neurocardiogenic syncope. I have had this condition for nine years and have been bedridden for the last two years. When I lift my head, I pass out, having no blood pressure. I have seen the best doctors and am currently taking Tenormin, Zoloft, Florinef, and Proamatine.

I need NASA's help. I have two children and a husband, along with a community that wishes and prays that I will be able to walk one day. I am currently using a surgical compression device, which fits like a blood pressure machine over my legs and feet, raising my blood pressure, which helps, but I cannot walk in it. Could you please help me by making me a suit I could walk in? The hot summer months are my hardest days. If I had a suit with air in it, I could maybe walk around. I long to see my front yard and my community, trees, and the sky. I heard that NASA does research for their astronauts and their blood pressure.

I can have my doctors write you if need be.

Please help me to live again!

Thank you for your time.

Lynn Fox Adams, Alabama

Working with NASA

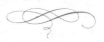

I began praying and thinking about how could I get out of this bed for my family and myself. I thought of NASA and how they work with blood pressures in space and on earth. So I wrote a letter and an e-mail to Daniel S. Golden for help. I told a friend about it, and that friend happened to know that Senator Sessions had a NASA representative in his office. She would only be there a few more days. That was God at work.

I called, and my friend also called. This resulted in working with a doctor from NASA, a Space Hall of Fame doctor who invented a flame-resistant space suit, Dr. Ralph Pelligra. He e-mailed Dr. Crawford and sent me a Velcro suit, which is a pressure suit. It had a big ball in the middle across my stomach. It Velcroed in sections: (1) ankle, (2) lower leg, (3) upper legs, and so on. Dr. Pelligra said that pressure around the stomach is more important than around the legs. It was very tight to bring the blood pressure up where it needed to be. The only problem was that when I took it off my blood pressure dropped drastically low.

When it arrived, my son helped me put it on, and we surprised my husband when he came home. I was sitting up for the first time in two years. It was a blessing because I was also able to sit up for Thanksgiving dinner that year, something I had not done for years. Although Ken would tell you it was a quick dinner—eating fast before I tired out—it was wonderful being with my family at the dinner table instead of being trapped in my dark, lonely room.

Dr. Pelligra had another idea to help me. He made me a suit filled with water; it had a pump that pumped water into a G suit. You see, with this condition, you can swim. Water takes over your blood pressure. I put on the suit, and Kenneth filled it up with water. It was quite heavy, but it did help. Dr. Pelligra talked with a paramedic while I first tried the suit out, so that way he could record my blood pressure readings accurately.

The suit did help my blood pressure rise. I also was told to take salt tablets, followed by eight ounces of water. The suit overall worked, but you had to drain it to take it off to use the restroom. One time my son had a friend call. My husband said, "Hang on. He's draining his mom's water." I know that must have sounded strange to a kid.

I also tried a diving suit. It was really tight and

helped with my blood pressure, and I could do a little more when I had it on. Keep in mind, I was still bedridden with an out-of-town doctor. In our old house, air conditioning came in the form of window units. In the hot summers, I stayed passed out. A dear friend of mine from our church helped us buy a mobile home. I wore the suit from NASA as we moved into a new home with central air conditioning; otherwise I would have had to go in an ambulance, which is very costly.

It was interesting working with the doctor from NASA, and it was too bad the suits didn't work out long-term. Dr. Pelligra taught me things that would help my condition, like raising the head of my bed five inches. He also told me to put blue ice on my body to help raise my blood pressure.

Dr. Pelligra has done so much research and studies on low blood pressure. He is the chief medical officer for NASA at the Ames Institute in California. It is important to have his explanation of seizures with dysautonomia because so many family members, once they hear *pseudo,* automatically say it is fake. Over the last decade I have talked with numerous sufferers of dysautonomia about how they too have lost family over this misunderstanding of pseudo-seizure.

Dr. Ralph Pelligra stated to me over the phone on August 27, 2008, that the word *pseudo* doesn't need to be used anymore. It is a word that is used when something other than the usual source is causing the health problem. Most seizures are caused by the brain, but with dysautonomia, the quick drop in blood pressure doesn't allow enough blood to get to the brain where it needs to be, causing a seizure. The seizure is real. From education and training and from my personal experience, Dr. Ralph Pelligra and I can both tell you they are very real. I hope this helps with the misunderstanding of seizures as far as dysautonomia is concerned. My own brother says I am not sick because of the word *pseudo*. My brother, not being a doctor, doesn't understand what *pseudo seizure* means. So I hope, with Dr. Pelligra's explanation, this will be cleared up. If you would like to read articles that Dr. Pelligra has written, simply Google his name, and you can read about his expert findings. I learned a lot about NASA and how they not only go to the moon but that they also help ordinary people. My many thanks to Dr. Rod Herring and Senator Jeff Sessions for their part in helping me find Dr. Ralph Pelligra. Working with NASA was a wonderful experience.

I wrote a poem about my experience with NASA.

Men walk on the moon,
As for me I would be satisfied
To be able to walk on earth!
But there is one thing I know,
Because I love the Lord
With all my heart,
And because I believe in Jesus,
Who died on a cross for me.
I will without a doubt
Be able to walk when I get to heaven!

Dear Lord,

Thank you for getting my letter to the president of NASA. Thank you for helping me learn more about blood pressures through Dr. Pelligra. Thank you for the opportunity to eat at the table with my family at Thanksgiving. That was truly a gift from you. Lord, I am asking you still to find me a doctor who can really help me get better and out of the bed. The days are so long and hard. The only thing that keeps me going is praying for others, listening to Larnell Harris and his gospel music about Jesus, and my friends, who encourage me daily. My husband and children help me. Thank you for sending Dr. Pelligra's expert findings on pseudo-seizures.

Dear Lord,

Today I received my Velcro suit. Please let it help me to feel better. Kenneth put it on me, and we surprised Ken when he arrived home. I was actually sitting up. Lord, your love is so mighty. I am leaning on you for guidance on the NASA suits.

JOURNAL ENTRY

Dear Lord,

It is exciting being able to sit up with the suit on. Although it is hot to wear, I can at least be up for short periods of time. Thank you, Lord, for those times. I love you, Lord, with all my heart, soul, and mind. Thank you for Kenneth, who helps me deal with my condition on a daily basis. He is so young but has a passion to help his mom feel better.

Thank You, Lord.
Lynn

JOURNAL ENTRY

Dear Lord,

I received another suit. This one has a pump that pumps water into a G suit. Kenneth helped me put it on in the hopes that I will be better. The suit did help, but it was awfully heavy being filled with water. And I also had to drain it and take it off to use the restroom. Lord, please help me and help my family as we strive to eliminate my suffering.

In a Nursing Home
at Thirty-Seven

In 1998 my health had become so bad that my doctor said I needed twenty-four-hour care, and my only option was to be placed in a nursing home. It wouldn't happen unless I had to go to the emergency room first. We called and told my parents the news. I was still struggling with my family's rejection. My mother drove to Alabama and tried to talk me out of it. What else could I do? My husband had to work, and we couldn't afford sitters. I was such a liability that no one would stay with me anyway.

When my mother arrived she headed for my room. She proceeded to yell at me, saying that it was ridiculous to go to a nursing home. She said, "You get up." That phrase always hurt me because all I wanted was to be up, and I tried often to do so. But since simply sitting up resulted in passing out, what could I do? Every time I passed out it took twenty-four hours to recover completely. Ken and I again tried to explain my condition to my parents like we had done for so many years. But they wouldn't listen. My mom still yelled at me.

The Bible states that if you have explained something to someone a number of times and they still do not understand, then call on someone from your church to come over and help.

> If your brother sins against you go and show him his fault, just between the two of you. If he listens to you, you have won your brother over. But if he will not listen, take one or two others along, so that every matter may be established by the testimony of two or three witnesses. If he refuses to listen to them, tell it to the church; and if he refuses to listen even to the church, treat him as you would a pagan or a tax collector.
>
> Matthew 18:15–17, NIV

So that's just what I did. I called someone from our church to come over and help explain my condition to my parents. He immediately came over and tried to reason with my mother that I was really sick. She said, "Yes, she is sick in the head."

Instead of leaning on God, I let her get me upset. I asked him to tell her to leave; I couldn't take the abuse anymore. That night I ended up being hauled off in an ambulance, which resulted days later in being placed in a nursing home. My minister, Ron, told me, "Lynn, you are here as a result of your parents. You cannot continue to see them if they are hurting you to the point that it affects your health."

I still loved my mom. But not having her support during the most difficult time in my life when I was taken away from my husband and two sweet children was almost unforgivable. I would have to go to God multiple times before I could come to terms with that.

The first day in the nursing home was the hardest day of my life. *Hard, difficult, depressing, awful*—those words aren't enough to describe how I felt when I arrived. All I could think about was that I had to get one more look at the sun and feel the breeze on my face. My physician said I needed twenty-four-hour care for the next several years until a new drug or suit was made to help people with my condition. Maybe I would remain there the rest of my life. I didn't know.

When they took me out of the ambulance, still on the stretcher, I can remember the paramedics looking at me and commenting on how young I was to be going to a nursing home, only thirty-seven years of age. As they took me out of the ambulance, I looked up at the beautiful blue sky and said, "Wait a moment." I asked the paramedics to let me lay there for just a few moments to feel the sun and wind on my face because I didn't know how long it would be until I felt them again. I could see tears welling up in one of the paramedic's eyes.

All of a sudden, two doors swung open, and an

awful smell came out. I looked around. The people there looked so depressed and out of it. The walls were plain. I remember thinking they needed to be painted a pretty color to brighten the place. I thought, *Oh Lord, how will I make it here without my husband and children? What will happen to them?* There were so many things running through my mind at the time. I certainly knew God was the only one who could help me.

I was taken to room 412. There was another lady there, my roommate, who did not respond to anything or anyone. My friend Linda was with me. She began to cry; I began to cry. The stretcher was placed beside my nursing home bed, and my roommate moved around so that I could just fit in. I was then lifted from the stretcher to the bed.

I remember my hands holding tightly to the stretcher sides; I didn't want to be put in that bed. The bed they were placing me in was very old, and I knew once I was put there that was where I would stay. I would stay for days, weeks, months, maybe years. I continued holding tightly to the ambulance stretcher, hoping it was all just a bad dream. Linda grabbed my hand, and, together with Ken, I was able to let go so that the paramedics could lift me into the other bed.

Boy was I right. The bed was hard, and the railing on it was pulled up so I would not fall out. It felt like jail bars. The railing was rusted; the bed was so old you had to hand-crank it. There was a curtain between my roommate and me that was mildewed green. I looked around the room and noticed that the ceiling above was discolored where it had leaked during a rain. Most of the blinds were missing. The walls needed painting so badly. I looked around again. I tried to find something good about the room but couldn't.

I thought, *No wonder my roommate is unresponsive.* No radio, no television, dirty walls, leaky ceilings—Linda and I were both sobbing at this point. Linda had brought some posters that the "Girls in Action" had given me from my church. I asked her to put them on the walls. I said, "Cover the walls and the ceiling. Jesus needs to shine here." Linda stood on my bed and put some on the ceiling so that when I was lying flat I would have something to look at.

Soon, my pastor, Ron, came into the room. He ran to me, and we hugged and sobbed together. My husband was trying to be strong for me, but I could tell he was upset. I thought, *Lord, I do not belong here. Help me!*

I knew that when I was at home I could no longer take care of myself. That meant I couldn't bathe, get my medication, or fix my lunch. My husband and children tried their best to take care of me, but my husband had to work, and my children were young and in school. I knew, physically, I needed to be in the nursing home. But emotionally, the only time you need to be in a nursing home is when your mind is gone. Now that I was in the nursing home, I wanted some other option, any option.

There was a lady in the adjoining room yelling,"

Help! Help!" over and over again. There I was. I didn't want to look at anything, or listen to anyone, or smell anything. That was the first time I had ever wished I could lose my senses. I didn't want to feel those railings that were pulled up on my bed. I didn't want to see, hear, feel, or smell, and later I would find out I sure didn't want to taste, not the nursing home food anyway.

When I was working and driving, I used to drive by the nursing home. I always thought it was a sad place; I couldn't even look at it. Now here I was, at age thirty-seven, living in it.

Linda had to leave, and Ken was getting ready to leave too. I couldn't bear to see him leave. I begged him to take me home with him. I can remember grabbing his wrist and hanging on for dear life. But we both knew he couldn't stay, and I couldn't leave. Later, after everyone left, I began to pray. "Dear Lord, help me! Heal me soon! I believe in your Word, and it says if you believe it will happen. I can't stay here a day, much less who knows how long. Lord, help me. Carry me, Lord! I need your love. In Jesus Christ's name, Amen." I then reached for my Bible and read. That was the only thing that got me through. The Bible is the most important book that was ever written. We forget that at times.

"Hear my cry, O God; listen to my prayer, from the ends of the earth I call to you, I call as my heart grows faint; lead me to the rock that is higher than I" (Psalm 61:1–2, NIV). The scripture says, "From the ends of the earth I call to you." Boy, was that true.

I felt like I was at the end of the earth, so far away from my family and friends. It also says, "As my heart grows faint," and it was surely faint.

"And we know that in all things God works for the good of those who love him, who have been called according to his purpose" (Romans 8:28, NIV). I prayed, "Lord, I know I have a purpose here. It is your will, your purpose. Lord, your Word says in all things God works for the good of those who love him. I love you with all my heart, soul, and mind." I needed something good to happen to me. At the time I didn't know what the good could possibly be. But later I would find out.

"Trust in the Lord with all your heart and lean not on your own understanding; in all your ways acknowledge him, and he will direct your paths" (Proverbs 3:5, NIV). I prayed again. "Lord, I am trusting in you with all my heart. I am glad I am not leaning on my understanding, because I do not understand. I am very weak physically. I do trust in you, Lord. After all, they can take away my material things—my family, my car, my money, my job—but no one can take you out of my heart. No one can take you away."

JOURNAL ENTRY

Dear Lord,

I haven't been in the nursing home long, but it seems like an eternity. I will focus on helping my roommate instead of myself. I believe you mean for us as Christians to put you first. And this lady needs you in her life desperately. Guide me and lead me to work for you and only you.

Lynn

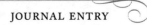

JOURNAL ENTRY

Dear Lord,

This place is so bad. They are not taking care of my roommate. They never check on her, and she cannot push the button for help. I will start pushing the button for her. I told them she needed a bath and to be fed. Oh Lord, I long for a hot cup of drinkable coffee. The food here is awful. It is not edible, and the dishes are dirty; the coffee is cold and bitter. I see the nurses walking by with a hot cup of coffee. They make it in their lounge. Lord, I am hungry, dirty. Won't someone help me? I am so sick physically, but I have Jesus in my heart. I will feed myself on your Word. But I cannot let my roommate go hungry. I have people come to see me and help me, but she doesn't. Lord, please send us some help.

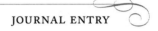

JOURNAL ENTRY

Dear Lord,

Thank you for my father-in-law. He bought me a laptop computer. I have found so many people

searching for help and acceptance with dysautonomia. I called the president of the dysautonomia
foundation and told her I wanted to be the support coordinator. She said, "Yes, we need some
help." I began to listen to people from the Internet and how they suffered. I printed out forty
pages of desperate people asking for help. One
man who called me needing my help and encour-
agement came from Blakely, Georgia, to meet me
in person. It was nice to see a face with a name.
Thank you, Lord, for using me for your glory.
Give me the strength to continue to help others.

Lynn

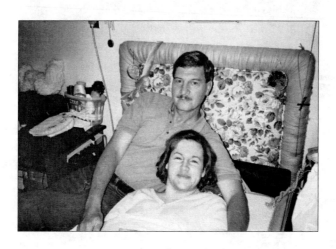

Miracle in Room 412

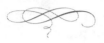

Ken brought my children to see me. Tricia was fourteen, and Kenneth was only ten years old. Tricia ran out of the room crying, "You can't leave my mom here!" I wanted so much to run after her, to tell her everything was going to be okay. I wanted to tell her I was coming home, but I couldn't do that. That wasn't true. Kenneth just stood there. He looked so sad. I prayed. "Heavenly Father, give me strength to be brave for my children. Help them, Lord, to understand and not to suffer. Help Ken to be able to take over as their physical mom, to do the things they need to have done. I know I can't be at home with my children, but I can certainly pray for them, Lord, so I am praying for them tonight. Help Tricia. I do not want her to hurt or be sad. Help Kenneth too. He is so young, and I'm concerned about him. Give him the love he needs through Ken and our church family. God, put people in his life that he needs. I love my family; please do not let this hurt them. I love you, Lord. In Jesus Christ's name, Amen."

After Ken and the kids left, I talked with God again. It suddenly seemed God was all I had. Little did I know, he was all I needed. The only noise I heard that night was the screaming of other patients. It was awful. One other thing I learned was that joy does come in the morning! After all the noise at night, it was rather peaceful early in the morning.

"For his anger lasts only a moment, but his favor lasts a lifetime; weeping may remain for a night, but rejoicing comes in the morning" (Psalm 30:5, NIV). Thank you, Lord, for the morning. For me, joy came the next day because I focused on God, not my situation.

I knew I could lie there, kick and scream, and feel sorry for myself, or I could serve God. I could even become angry at God for letting me be there. But I chose to serve the Lord. I resolved to tell others about Jesus Christ, and I wanted to start with my unresponsive roommate.

She was eighty-eight years old and had no teeth, no legs, and hardly any hair. She lay in a bed that looked like a coffin. It had a mattress that blew up. She didn't speak or open her eyes or move. I could hardly see her because of the curtain between us. Her bed faced the other direction from mine.

I started talking to her. I read her the Bible, played her gospel music on my tape player, and together we worshiped the Lord. After several weeks of saying Jesus's name to her she began to make some noise. I continued to share God's love with her. Even though we both lay flat and couldn't see each other, it didn't matter. We were worshiping the Lord. My roommate started to smile and say, "Jesus!" Praise the Lord! Even though she had nothing else, she had Jesus. The nurses and aides started to come in the room to see what had happened to her. "She is awake!" one stated.

"For where two are three come together in my name there am I with them" (Matthew 18:20, NIV). She and I were two gathered together praising God's name. I had the aides move our room around so we could see each other a little. We sang hymns and prayed, and I read the Bible to her. I would have never dreamed I would be best friends with an eighty-eight-year-old lady who couldn't do anything. After several weeks she had sparks in her eyes as if she had a reason to live. She just needed Jesus's love. She would often cry at night to go home. I would tell her that her real home was in heaven with God. Then we would sing "Jesus Loves Me" all night long.

One time we got so loud that one of the nurses asked us to be quiet. That didn't stop us. I wasn't about to make a lady who hadn't made a sound for over a year be quiet, especially when we were praising the Lord. I wondered why it was okay for people to yell when they were out of it, but not okay to sing when they were with it. I didn't know what was going on in the other parts of the world, but in room 412, we were praising God.

Eventually other residents began to come into our room and sing with us. My roommate began to clap along with the gospel music. That was a miracle. I asked my husband to bring a big balloon and some bubbles to the nursing home. My son and I would throw the balloon at her, and after a while, she started to hit it back to us, even though one of her hands was mangled from a stroke. She would laugh and hit the balloon back and forth, and she began to get stronger. I was amazed at what God did. Could this be the same lady, the lady who had been dying and in an unconscious state? It showed me what the love of Christ can do if we spread it around. It can make a difference in someone's life.

I asked the nurse's assistant why no one came to see her. She said, "We don't know why, but she hasn't had a visitor in quite a while." I asked the nurse to find out if she had any children. Later I was told she had a daughter and some grandchildren and great-grandchildren. They lived right in the same town as the nursing home. I resolved to call her daughter as soon as my phone was hooked up.

My roommate didn't have anything, so I asked several of my friends to buy her a few things: soap, a gown, clip-on earrings, and a bow for her hair. I asked the nursing assistant to bathe her. She did, and she put on her pretty new gown and her big clip-on earrings and put the bow in her hair. I asked the nursing assistant to hand her a mirror so she could see herself. My roommate took one look at herself in the mirror and smiled the biggest smile I had ever seen. It was a true miracle. I will never forget the joy in her face as she looked at herself.

I asked our minister of music, John Leland, if he would bring a microphone and speaker so she could hear me read the Bible to her better. The day he brought that microphone and speaker was an amazing day. My roommate held the microphone in her mangled hand the best she could and sang "Jesus Loves Me." It didn't matter that she didn't have teeth or couldn't speak well. With the sounds she made, I could tell what she was trying to sing. I could tell from her sweet spirit that Jesus was in her heart. To this day, that is still the sweetest sound I have ever heard.

Look at what God had done. He took a lady who hadn't opened her eyes in over a year, and she was sitting up singing. What a joy! I finally got in touch with her daughter, but she said she didn't have a car. She stated that the last time she had come to the nursing home her mother didn't know her and didn't open her eyes. I told her she had to come because her mother was sitting up singing and smiling and praising the Lord. Her daughter did not believe me, but she said she would come.

Several days later her daughter and granddaughter came. When they entered the room they couldn't believe their eyes. She was dressed with a bow in her hair, had earrings on, and was sitting up and smiling. Her daughter said, "It's a miracle. I have my mom back." Her daughter walked over to me and said, "Lynn, thank you. I have been praying every day for someone to help her."

I said, "I mostly read Psalm 23 to her and played gospel music." She began to cry, saying Psalm 23 was her mother's favorite Bible verse and that gospel was her favorite music. We praised the Lord that day, and my roommate enjoyed one more day with her daughter and granddaughter. Right before Christmas she became sick, having had another stroke, and she was sent to the hospital. She remained in the hospital for a week, which seemed like an eternity for me; I missed her. While she was gone, I had another roommate who yelled to go to Dallas, Texas, all night long. One of my friends asked me how my night was, and I told him to buy my new roommate a ticket to Dallas.

When my first roommate returned she yelled because she was so happy to see me. We sang and praised God all night and began to make plans for Christmas. The next day three nurses came to get her. They were moving her to another section of the nursing home. She began to cry as they moved her bed, and she reached for me. I couldn't sit up or get up, so I tried to reach my arm through the rails of my bed to hold her hand. She screamed while I cried. As they rolled her out and she was screaming, I swung my foot over my railing and showed her the man on the bottom of my foot. I saw one last smile as she was rolled away.

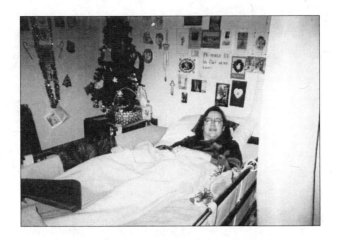

We were each unable to leave our beds or rooms, so we didn't get to see each other again. Two and a half months later she died. I can honestly say I will never forget her. She forever changed my life, for she taught me that no matter what situation you are in, you can always share Jesus's love.

"The Lord gives strength to his people, the Lord blesses his people with peace" (Psalm 29:11, NIV). I have truly lived this verse.

Once a private room became available I was able to move into it. After I moved in I got my friend Karen to help me make a "Heaven's Hotel Hallelujah Bulletin Board," inspired by my late roommate and based on a song we used to sing, "Heaven's Hotel Hallelujah." On it, I had pictures of people, and with the pictures, people wrote how and when they had been saved. It was truly a blessing. I feel we need to share our testimonies more often.

On the bulletin board, I also had the steps on

how to become saved. After several months and a lot of witnessing, two nursing assistants were saved. Praise the Lord!

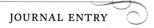

JOURNAL ENTRY

Dear Lord,

Thank you for saving my two new friends. I am glad they now have Jesus in their hearts. Thank you to Ken and Shannon Vickery for singing my roommate and me the song "Heaven's Hotel Hallelujah," which inspired the bulletin board on my room wall. Thank you for blessing me. I am glad my old roommate is no longer suffering but with you in heaven.

JOURNAL ENTRY

Dear Lord,

Here I am, in a nursing home during Thanksgiving. Gary brought me a sausage biscuit from Hardee's. It was so good. Dorinda brought me some of their lunch. I sure do miss being able to sit at the table with my family. I will never get those moments back. I hope people realize how blessed they are to be able to sit together and pray together. Lord, just help me to shine for you. I have a Bible storybook about Mary, Joseph, and Baby Jesus, and I read it to residents all the time. Help them learn to know Jesus in their own way. I love you.

Lynn

JOURNAL ENTRY

Dear Lord,

Oh, how I long for a hot cup of coffee. I decided to make a big sign, and on it, I drew a cup of hot coffee and put, "I will buy for a dollar." I held it up every time anyone walked by. Linda brought me some Pop-Tarts for breakfast. I decided if I wanted them hot, I would have to do it myself. So I reached for my blow dryer and blew it on the Pop-Tart until it was hot.

Lynn

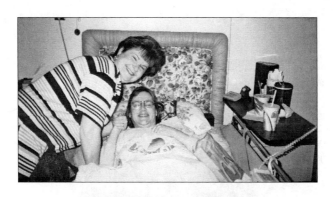

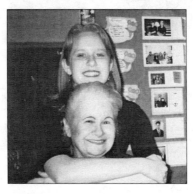

My Angel in a Baseball Cap

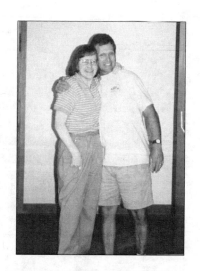

One October day in 1998, during football season, I was stuck in the nursing home and couldn't see my kids in the band. I looked up from my bed and saw a man with flowers! I thought, *Who is this man?* He walked in and handed me some bulldog carnations and introduced himself as Randy. I thought, *Do I know him? Why is he here?*

He said, "I go to First Baptist Church, and I also work with the Opelika High School Band. I know your daughter, Tricia, and I would love to take pictures of her at the next game.

I said, "Great! Thank you." I thought it was nice of a stranger to bring me flowers to cheer me up. Little did I know, Randy and I were not strangers.

We had a spiritual relationship that started way before we met. Randy said, "The Lord laid it on my heart to pray for you, Lynn, in 1994." I could feel tears in my eyes because, on August 4, 1994, I collapsed. That was the last day I worked or drove a car or even walked without fainting. Since then, I had been mostly bedridden. In 1994 I shared my illness with only a few close friends. How could he have known who I was, much less what was going on in my life? As we talked, I felt like we had known each other for years. That day started the first day of a wonderful friendship.

Randy and I gathered there in the nursing home. I had plenty of visitors; some just wanted to see the young girl in the nursing home. Few prayed with me. Most came to sit down and tell me their problems. Jesus didn't come into the world to answer our problems. He is the answer to our problems. I found that this is a very lonely world. Everyone is too busy to listen to one another's needs. I listened. What choice did I have? There I was, completely bedridden and unable to leave.

God heard my prayers and sent an eternal friend, Randy, someone who longed to read God's Word and pray just like I wanted to. Randy has helped me through not only what was a physical battle, but he also helped me keep my spiritual flame burning. I was so sick that I could not see to read my Bible at times, so he would read it for me. When my voice was too weak to pray, he prayed for me.

Several weeks later I had some problems with my room. When it rained the ceiling leaked, and it soaked the ceiling tile. Then the ceiling collapsed on me. I often prayed to be able to go outside to see God's beauty, to feel the sun and the breeze. After the ceiling collapsed on me twice I began to wonder if it rained in on top of my head so I could feel some of God's nature like I had prayed for.

Then fire ants fell out of the ceiling on top of me and my roommate. Now I could enjoy a good picnic, except I had the ants without any of the good food. After telling the nurse several times about the ants to no avail, she finally listened the day I started yelling for her. That day I had taped the ants to my bed. Previously, she had sent a maintenance man in to look for them, but he could never find any because they were dropping from the ceiling.

When my friend Jim walked in, it was raining on both sides of my bed, and he heard me crying for coffee. He stood there and just watched it rain in on me. The assistant administrator finally decided to move me into another room so they could fix the ceiling and get rid of the ants. I was taken to room 422. After being up all night listening to people yell, "Help me," having the rain come in, and the fire ants biting me, I was very tired. The social worker came to the room I was in and said, "I'd like to get you lunch since you have had a rough day. How about a steak?" Then she said, "Give me some money!" I guess she thought that I didn't know the rules of the nursing home: no money allowed. Boy, by that time, she had my mouth watering for a steak and baked potato.

After she left I thought, *Lord, just send me some lunch that I can eat.* The nursing home food was not edible. Randy, my angel in a baseball cap, showed up. He said, "I finally found you. I know you are tired and hungry. I would love to buy you lunch! What about a steak and a baked potato?" I started laughing and explained to him what had happened with the social worker. After he left to pick up my lunch, I had tears in my eyes because I knew God sent him so that I would not be hungry. "Therefore I tell you, do not worry about your life, what you will eat or drink; or about your body, what you will wear. Is not life more important than food, and the body more important than clothes?" (Matthew 6:25, NIV). Randy came back shortly with some bottled colas, a steak, and a baked potato.

Randy was not only my angel, but he was also a servant for our Lord! There were so many people who needed Jesus's love and to know him. I was too sick physically. It became impossible for me to read the Bible to so many people. God knew I needed help, and Randy was that help. Randy forever touched my life. I would pray, "Dear Lord, I am hungry," and Randy would bring food. He brought cokes when I was thirsty, bubblegum when I was in pain, chocolate when I was nauseated, and towels when I was dirty.

Randy and I read Scripture, studied God's Word, prayed, and rejoiced in his glory. I was like a car without gas; I needed to have my spirit refilled so I could continue to share about Jesus. Randy was the pump that supplied that spirit.

"Since we live by the Spirit, let us keep in step with the Spirit" (Galatians 5:25, NIV). Although I could not walk physically, I could renew my spirit and keep in step. It was difficult because I could not attend church, which helps to keep us in step with the Spirit. I loved my time alone with the Lord. I spent so many nights praying, reading his Word, and listening to praise music. I truly began to have a closer relationship with the Lord. That was awesome, but I needed others to help me learn and grow in the Spirit. Spiritually, I felt like I was on a treadmill, going in the same direction over and over. When Randy and I prayed together and talked about God and read his Word, it was like being on an escalator. The definition of escalator is "a moving stairway on an endless belt." The longer we spent time in God's Word, the more my step with the Spirit grew. We were lifted to heaven on an endless belt where God was stepping for us. We just had to be in tune with God's spirit. God longs for his time with us.

At Easter, Randy asked me to teach his Sunday school class by video. I prayed about it. People did need to hear about all the things God has blessed them with that they take for granted like being able to sit up, walk, attend church, and be with their families. I was excited because it would be almost like I was attending Sunday school, something I had longed for. That Sunday school lesson would become the most meaningful lesson I had ever taught. The things I taught I had learned from God. I had lived the words I spoke through Jesus Christ.

Randy enriched my life so much that year visiting me and helping me weekly. I am so thankful I did not turn away the stranger at my nursing home door that day. I thank God for Randy, "my angel in a baseball cap."

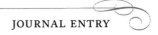

JOURNAL ENTRY

Dear Lord,

Thank you for all the help Randy has given me, especially since he could come in the day time when my husband couldn't. My husband came at night, but the doors were locked at 9:00 p.m., so our visits were short. Thank you, Lord, for Linda, who washes my clothes weekly. She is a blessing to me. God, you are so good.

Dear Lord,

Thank you for sending Jim Allen with a hot cup of coffee. The ceiling fell on me, and it actually rained in my room. Ants were also eating me. I am thankful something was finally done with those two problems. You are good to me, for you sent me help when I needed it. Thank you, my Lord and Savior.

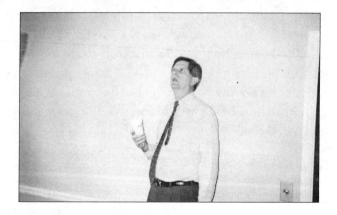

A Light in a Very Dark Place

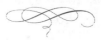

It was right before Christmas, and the "Girls in Action" from my church had brought me a Christmas tree with ornaments that had Bible verses on them. There were also angels and other wooden ornaments on the tree. I had a friend hang a big cross with tinsel on my wall by my bed. Residents came often to see my decorated room. I read them the story of Mary, Joseph, and Baby Jesus.

It was around this time that there was a lady at the nursing home I became close to. She suffered from cerebral palsy. She could not speak, but she seemed to have something to say; I could tell. She would wheel by my room, slow down, look at me, and smile. That smile, even without teeth, was beautiful. After some weeks she wheeled herself into my room. She made noises as if she were telling me something important. I read the story of Jesus to my new friend every day for a week. She began to learn how to say "Jesus." I was thrilled.

One day I saw her darting very quickly up and down in the hall in her wheelchair. This went on for hours. A doctor, nurses, and aides were all chasing her, and she was crying. I pushed my call light and asked what was wrong with her. The nurse said, "They have to move her to a semiprivate room." She had always had a private room.

I said, "Send her to my room." When she entered I asked her what was wrong. She kept trying to speak, making loud noises. I told her, "You are so tired. You have been up all day crying. Go into your room." I told her when the door was open she could still see me from her bed because her room was opposite mine. I told her we would say our prayers together every night, and that it was going to be okay. I handed her an angel off my Christmas tree and told her to take it and to hang it on her bed. I told her I would look out for her, and so would the angel. "Jesus loves you, and so do I." She wiped the tears from her eyes with her mangled hand, then smiled and went right into her new room. She leaned over her railing, and I could see her. She smiled and was okay. Every night we sang "Jesus Loves Me" and prayed.

I began to spend one-on-one time with her. She learned how to sing "Jesus Loves Me" and "This Little Light of Mine." I asked a friend of mine to check a children's Bible storybook out of our church library. We read a story every day. My experience teaching preschool at church for years came in handy at the nursing home.

I called the state and asked my friend's social worker for some materials to work with her. She was smart but trapped in a body that couldn't speak. Both the state and her social worker said my friend was too old for materials, but I didn't believe that. I had people gather some larger crayons, big balloons, and bubbles. I taught her how to color; she did wonderful staying in the lines. Eventually I taught her how to write her name. She was even able to type her name on my computer using the end of a pencil. My new friend came in my room with a Sears catalog and showed me a picture of a computer just like mine. I knew what she was saying. She wanted one too. That's how smart she was. She had never had a chance to learn, having been in a nursing home her whole life. She didn't know what churches, restaurants, or houses were.

One day I was struggling with longing to go home. I was crying, wanting just to go home and be with my family. I was very upset. She wheeled into my room and grabbed my hand and comforted me. I told her I wanted to go home. She looked at me like, "What in the world are you talking about?" At least I knew what home was and the world outside.

Here was a lady who would never have a husband or children or a life in the world outside. She stayed indoors, never going out. She had never seen a waterfall, mountains, a river, or a stream. How awful that would be! How blessed people are to be able to see God's beauty!

She had a pattern for making dogs out of yarn; she sold her creations for five dollars. One day she brought me a dog she had made and fussed for her five-dollar bill. I was laughing because I didn't order one.

She often stole my disinfectant spray and took it

to her room. Randy always supplied me with disinfectant spray, but she would come into my room and take it for herself. Once, she asked me to call Randy to bring her some spray. I said, "No. You have learned how to say his name, so you can call him." I dialed the phone, and the answering machine came on. Now, you try and explain that to someone like her; she heard his voice, but he wasn't there! She looked at me like I was out of my mind.

I was upset that the cardiologist I had seen in the hospital had not come to see me while I was in the nursing home. It had been months, and I kept calling the office. What I didn't realize was that the doctor who put me in the nursing home had to give permission for Dr. Davis to treat me, and he had not. So I talked with someone from the state and told them my problem. I wanted Dr. Davis, the cardiologist, to come see me. Maybe one day I would be able to sit up and go home. I couldn't imagine staying in the nursing home much longer.

This call resulted in Dr. Davis finally coming to see me. He had been studying my condition and had a few ideas he thought would help. One was a device with pedals like a bicycle that screwed to the end of my bed. He told me to ride the bike for five minutes several times a day. So I put my friend in charge of my exercising. I asked her to tell me when five minutes was up. I would ask her, and she would hold up three fingers. I would ask again later, and she would hold up three fingers. Then again, and guess what? Three fingers! I really got my exercise.

To this day she still calls me from the nursing

home. Although I don't understand what she is saying, I listen and talk back. She still knows how to sing "Jesus Loves Me" and "This Little Light of Mine." What a blessing she has been to me.

I realized, through her, how blessed even I was. I had gotten the chance to live outside of those nursing home walls. She would never know those things, and that reminded me daily how grateful I should be.

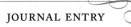

JOURNAL ENTRY

Dear Lord,

Here I am still in the nursing home. You know my heart and how I long to go home. But there are people here who need to know Jesus! I love you with all my heart, so use me no matter what the sacrifice. I pray the pacemaker that Dr. Davis plans on putting in me will help me be able to sit up. Help Tricia and Kenneth while I am in the nursing home. Let them know that I love them and want to be with them. Give them your love. Help them to grow up and become strong Christians for you, for you are so good.

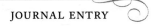

JOURNAL ENTRY

Dear Lord,

Today Tricia is dancing at the arts festival. I wish and long to be there to see her dance. Oh Lord, people here need to know you. So many people just die and die alone. When I find out about someone dying without anyone with them, I call my church and have someone come and sit with them and read them the Bible and pray with them. Lord, continue to use me for your glory. It is very hard to be here, but I know you have a purpose, and I know one day I will sit up. Love you.

JOURNAL ENTRY

Dear Lord,

I have passed out several times today. But this afternoon, as I turned on my computer, I had dozens of messages from people who were suffering from dysautonomia. Help me help them, Lord. They need you in their lives first of all.

JOURNAL ENTRY

Dear Lord,

Today is Sunday again, and the pain of my not being able to attend church with my family is so great. I hurt for that opportunity. So please comfort me from my head to my toes. I long for my husband and children. I long to be a part of their lives. I can never get the past back. Heal me, Lord. I want so much to be able to sit up, and I believe I will. Love you.

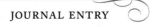

JOURNAL ENTRY

Dear Lord,

Today was a bad day. But, as usual, you make me stronger through my difficulties. It teaches me to lean on you 100% and not myself. Today I went over to the surgical center by ambulance. It felt so good to feel the wind outside, even if it was just for a moment. I pray for Dr. Davis as he strives to help me sit up and go home.

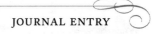

JOURNAL ENTRY

Dear Lord,

Wow! I had a very special guest today. Judy Colley surprised me by bringing Elizabeth Elliott, one of my favorite authors and speakers, to meet me. I love her radio show and books. She gave me two autographed books. I just hate that I talked the whole time and didn't let her talk more. I admire her and how she has handled her struggles. Thank you, Lord, for such a special day.

JOURNAL ENTRY

Dear Lord,

I long for the simple things: to take a shower, to go outside and see the birds, to feel the wind or rain. But please do not let it rain in my room anymore. I long to be with my family. I believe and know, dear Lord, that you will one day help me sit up without passing out.

One thing that was exciting today was that I heard Kenneth play the trombone over the phone. He is talented. I miss him so much.

JOURNAL ENTRY

Dear Lord,

Today is Mother's Day, and I am very sad. I just want my mother to accept and love me. I also want to be at home with my children. I feel like they are growing up without me in their lives. The only thing I can do for them is pray. I long to be in church with them. I am sad today. Lord, make me feel better.

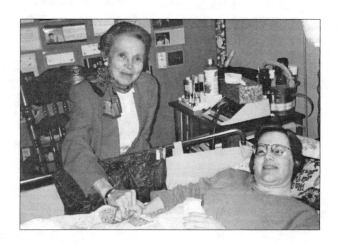

The Devotional at
the Nursing Home

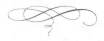

On February 2, 1999, I was asked to give the devotional in the activities room for the residents. Even though I could not sit up, I decided I could still tell people about Jesus and his love. People in the nursing home needed some hope.

I had to be wheeled down to the activities room in my bed with my suit on and ice covering me. A friend of mine went from room to room telling people, "Get up. Lynn is giving the devotional. You need to hear it." There was a lady who was still sleeping, but I especially wanted her to come because she spent most of her time wandering around saying, "I want to go home. Please take me home." She even offered people money to take her home, but her home was gone. My goal was to give the message that our real home is in heaven, not here on earth. I thought having this message come from someone who was living with them would make all the difference.

> Jesus replied, "If anyone loves me, he will obey my teachings. My Father will love him, and we will come to him and make our home with him."
>
> John 14:23, NIV

> Therefore we are always confident and know that as long as we are at home in the body we are away from the Lord. We live by faith, not by sight. We are confident, I say, and would prefer to be away from the body and at home with the Lord.
>
> 2 Corinthians 5:6–9, NIV

We had a full room. More than forty residents came because my friend had gone out and encouraged them to come. I told how our home was with Jesus Christ, our Lord, not in a house somewhere. I had a stick and a rose. I showed the stick and explained that the stick was how I was before I got saved—nothing special—and they passed the stick around to feel it. Then I explained how, after I accepted Jesus Christ as my Savior, I became a rose. I asked Jesus into my heart, and he saved me. I explained how Jesus died on the cross for our sins, and if we believe he rose again, we would be like a rose and be saved. The closer we get to God, the more beautiful our petals will be. They seemed to understand that.

I knew how they felt about wanting to go home, so I needed to share with them verses about hope. I asked them to put their hope in God, not things. In him our hearts rejoice, for we trust in his holy name.

May your unfailing love rest upon us O Lord, even as we put our hope in you.

Psalm 33:22, NIV

Find rest, O my soul, in God alone; my hope comes from him. He alone is my rock and my salvation; he is my fortress, I will not be shaken. My salvation and my honor depend on God; he is my Mighty rock and my refuge. Trust in him at all times O people; pour out your hearts to him, for God is our refuge.

Psalm 62:5–8, NIV

By the end of the devotional people were shouting with me, "My hope is in the Lord!" I kept repeating that with a loud voice until everyone was making a noise. Those who couldn't talk smiled and spoke in their own way. What a blessing it was to see so many disabled people thanking God in the midst of their circumstances.

While they were wheeling me out on my bed the lady who always cried to go home was walking out with her walker. She stopped me and said, "Lynn, I am not going to whine to go home anymore." She said her home was in heaven, and her hope was in the Lord! What a miracle. She had learned that her material home was not of importance. The nurses and her aides thanked me for that one.

I had ended the devotional by handing out Bibles because few had one. I not only handed them out to residents but also to some nurses. Some of the patients held onto their Bibles for hope even if they couldn't read. To this day there is a man in the nursing home who still carries his Bible in his wheelchair even though he doesn't know how to read. Most of them brought their Bibles to me to read to them. They put Bibles in hotel rooms but not nursing homes; that is not right, and I do not understand it.

Psalm 23 was a very popular and familiar passage to read.

This scripture was so popular during my stay at the nursing home because people were there to die. They were walking through the shadow of death. My goal was that they would accept Jesus so they could dwell in the house of the Lord forever.

Listen. We will either die young or old. The chances of us being in a place like the nursing home are great. Since I have lived through that already, let me give you some suggestions. Your eyesight will go, so it will be hard to read the Bible at all. Then your hearing will go, making it hard to hear someone else reading to you. So what we all need to do is memorize Bible verses and songs so that we do not lose sight of God while we are waiting for that escalator to take us to heaven.

JOURNAL ENTRY

Dear Lord,

Dr. Davis came today. Help him figure out a way to help me get out of the nursing home. He is caring and smart; use him for your glory. Dr. Davis told me he would never give up on me. That gave me comfort. He knew how I longed to be with my family at home. He began getting books and information and studying on my condition. He was willing to do anything. He seemed to be the doctor I had been praying for all along. Thank you, Lord. I love you with all my heart, soul, and mind.

JOURNAL ENTRY

Dear Lord,

I pray that the people of the nursing home will come to know you. Even if they suffer from a physical or mental condition, they can still know Jesus Christ. Use me to introduce him to them. Use me to help them learn about Jesus. I have to admit I think I have sung "Jesus Loves Me" about a thousand times since I have been here.

New Promises

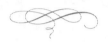

Dr. Crawford, my cardiologist in Montgomery, Alabama, was an hour away; she was the one who had put me in the nursing home to start with. Since Dr. Crawford lived out of town, she didn't have legal rights at the nursing home to treat me. So she asked Dr. Davis to treat me.

God worked it out for him to see me because Dr. Davis had only worked for Montgomery Cardiovascular for a brief time. If it had been a month later I wouldn't have found Dr. Davis. After he left the Montgomery practice he started his own cardiovascular practice in Opelika, Alabama, my own town. "If you believe, you will receive whatever you ask for in prayers" (Matthew 21:22, NIV).

Dr. Davis had a new plan. He put a heart monitor on me and found out I needed a permanent pacemaker. Our plan was to start overdosing me on a beta blocker. Finally, a doctor was not afraid to try and help me, to try things that hadn't been tried before. He was the doctor I had prayed for. He believed in me and understood my condition. Thank you, Lord.

Around the time I found out I was going to have surgery, the Lord laid it on my heart to make some badges for people to wear that said, "I believe." God showed me over and over that if people would pray, they would receive what they have asked for in Jesus' name. When God first laid it on my heart to make the badges, I did not listen. I mentioned it to several people, but no one wanted to help. Some even said, "You know, Lynn, you have been sick a long time. You probably won't ever walk." I was to have surgery in March, and it was already February. I didn't obey. I developed an infection in my chest that stayed for over a month, and I couldn't have the surgery. It was only when I finally surrendered and agreed to do the Lord's will that I was finally healed and able to reschedule the surgery.

All throughout my journal and my Bible I had written, "I believe." I knew God wanted me to make those badges so people would believe, and later it would be revealed in God's time. Two days before the surgery, I was finally working on the badges. On them, I put a rainbow because the rainbow represents God's covenant promise. Also, I felt like Noah must have, with people thinking I was being ridiculous wanting people to wear badges. In Genesis chapters 6–8, Noah obeys God even though people treat him badly and think he's crazy.

In the middle of the badge was a gold cross because prayers will not be answered until you have surrendered your life to Jesus Christ and are saved. I also put two scriptures on the badges: "Then Jesus told his disciples a parable to show them that they should always pray and never give up" (Luke 18:1, NIV). "Be joyful always, pray continually; give thanks in all circumstances, for this is God's will for you in Christ Jesus" (Thessalonians 5:16–18, NIV).

As I was finishing, Randy came into my room. I immediately said, "I need your help." I sent him to buy laminate sheets. We copied and cut out thirty badges. He handed them out to the staff, and I handed the rest to my family, friends, my pastor, and others. It only took a day for people to start asking for more. Tricia's friends all wanted one. People at the church wanted them too. We had not made enough.

The next day was it: my long-awaited surgery. As I was being put in the ambulance to go to the hospital, I got another look at the sky and felt the wind on my face. Thank you, Lord. At the hospital, my pastor came in the room to pray with Ken and me before surgery. He was wearing his badge, and so was my cousin Sandy. All I could think about was whether I could go home after surgery. Would the pacemaker help me enough to send me back home to my family? I knew that the Lord would help me in his time. I also knew if I believed, had faith, prayed, and never gave up, God could heal me.

After the surgery I spent the night at the hospital

then was sent back to the nursing home. It was so hard for me to go back there, but with God I would make it and continue to pray for healing. Sandy spent the night and helped me get settled back into my room. Over the next several months, Dr. Davis planned to try beta blockers for my condition.

In the nursing home they had me on an air-inflated bed because at times they had to cover me with ice to raise my blood pressure. As I was lying on the half-inflated bed, an elderly lady was trying to get in bed with me. She kept saying, "Why are you in my bed?" I kept telling her that it wasn't her bed or her room, that she'd have to go. There sure wasn't enough room for her in my bed. It was bad when I would rather stay in a hospital than where I was living. The hospital was like a hotel, and I missed it. I especially missed the mattress and the privacy.

While I was in the nursing home, there were residents who often yelled, "Help me!" and I learned to teach them to say, "Lord, help me." Another challenge I had at the nursing home was bathing in that pink, six-inch tub that was two inches deep. Try to picture someone who can't sit up bathing from two inches of cold water. Would you start with your feet or face? Of course I started with my face, down to my feet. It was such a challenge. Try lying flat and washing your face. It is pretty much impossible. One thing I longed for was a hot shower while standing up all by myself. If you take a hot shower, then for goodness' sake, sing while you are in the shower, shout if you want to. Just thank the Lord.

Ken always visited me on Friday nights. That was our time together. I knew it was hard for Ken to see me at the nursing home, but he came anyway. He would also surprise me with a hot cup of coffee and some donuts. Every time he came I wished I could leave with him, and he wished it too. He was raising the kids alone and juggling two jobs; he was quite busy and didn't get to come see me as much as he wanted to.

Tricia came to visit and was learning to drive. Kenneth was so much younger. Ken would drop him off, and he would stay with me for hours. At times he helped me wash my hair and cooked things in the microwave for me. The whole time I was in the nursing home was so difficult. It was hard on all of us.

JOURNAL ENTRY

Dear Lord,

I had the surgery. I hope it will help me. Dr. Davis said I needed it. I pray it will help me sit up and feel better. I believe that with you, God, anything can happen. I long to sit up; help me, Lord. I have been trapped in this bed too long. I love you.

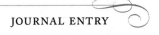

JOURNAL ENTRY

Dear Lord,

I am so thankful for my cousin Sandy. She came down to be here for my surgery because my parents and brother would not come. I enjoyed her, and we prayed for the hope that the pacemaker and medication would help me sit up and get out of the nursing home. I am thankful she knows me and believes in me. I am so glad her parents also love and believe in me. Uncle Hollis confronted my mom and told her how he had seen me sick in the hospital. But she still didn't accept it. I pray for my mom, dad, and brother, that they will learn what love is. As of now, they are turning against me. Lord, you know the truth and have a plan. I will get guidance from you.

My Darkest Day

Oh Lord, every day I prayed and spent time with you and believed I would eventually sit up. The scriptures tell us that if we have faith and believe, it will happen. "Ask and it will be given to you, seek and you will find; knock and the door will be opened to you. For everyone who asks receives; he who seeks finds; and to him who knocks, the door will be opened" (Matthew 7:7–8, NIV). It was July 1999 when I felt so desperate to leave the nursing home.

I noticed people had stopped wearing their badges after the surgery. I called everyone and told them not to give up. I told them that God had a plan and to keep wearing them. Dr. Davis began progressively overdosing me on a blood pressure medication. This was our hope that I would sit up. I started out on 80mg, then after six weeks 160mg, then 240mg.

After 240mg, I began to get sicker. I kept throwing up and felt very ill. I began to get dehydrated, but the nurses did nothing except tell me to eat. I kept explaining I was too nauseated. I felt different. I started to have a "give up" attitude. I could not bathe myself in God's Word; I couldn't see to read the Bible. I felt so bad physically that I did not want to live. I felt my hope fading away. How could I stay there away from my family? How could I continue to live in a nursing home? I kept telling everyone who visited to get me out of the nursing home, but no one could really help; only God could.

I e-mailed Dr. Davis and asked him when I would sit up. I told him I was sicker and was not able to eat or drink. He e-mailed me back, saying, "It is like a *Star Trek* episode. We are going where no man has gone before." He didn't know if I would ever sit up. I longed to sit up more and more each day. I prayed. I cried. I pleaded with God and everyone who came to see me.

I felt so trapped, locked up like I was in jail. But I do believe that if I had been in jail I would have been taken better care of. They wouldn't wash my hair or bring me water for a bath or empty my urinal. They were bringing the wrong medications at the wrong times. If I needed ice, the chest would be empty. I kept asking why I was there if they didn't listen or take care of me. They brought me meals that were cold and old-tasting, and I was so nauseated I couldn't eat them. My physical condition was getting worse, and I was getting depressed.

As weeks passed I became sicker. I begged them

to call Dr. Davis. Ken decided he would go to his office and talk to him about coming to see me. After all, the nursing home staff wouldn't call him and tell him how sick I was. So my sweet husband went to Dr. Davis's office and demanded to talk with him.

The staff kept making the comment that I wouldn't eat the food. When my pastor came I said, "You have got to get me out of here." I told all my friends who visited, "Get me out of here." I called Dr. Davis and cried, saying I had to see him before I ended up dead from dehydration. I didn't hear from him that day.

Since I felt no one would help, I decided to rescue myself. I kept thinking that if I could crawl out of my room and steal something, maybe they would put me in jail. Maybe I would at least get to see the sun and trees on my way to jail. I kept thinking that in jail I could get twenty-four-hour care, better food, and even a chance to go outside. I decided to plan an escape.

The maintenance man came in to fix the bathroom. He laid his hammer on my stand by my bed, and I hid it. I received a candle from a friend, and she had some matches, and I hid them. I decided to try to crawl off the bed late at night. If I kept my head lower than my feet, I would hopefully not pass out. After getting off the bed, I would crawl out the sliding glass door. I planned on going to the woods next door. I would probably not live long in the heat, but I wanted to be free. What could I lose? No one was listening, and if they were they couldn't do anything about it.

I would break free for at least several hours. I put the hammer, candle, matches, a drink, a towel, and some wet wipes in my pillowcase. It was one thirty a.m. The usual yelling of residents was going on, so I knew no one would hear me trying to escape. Out of the sliding glass door was a courtyard surrounded by rooms and brick walls, except one area to the right of my room. There was only a wooden fence. I would hammer at the bottom of the fence. Hopefully they would loosen up so I could crawl under, or I would dig my way out. I could only imagine the beautiful night and the sky, stars, and the fresh air. *Oh God, help me to be able to escape and see your beauty.*

I got my pillowcase and started working on lowering the bed rails. I had been behind those bed rails long enough; freedom was all I could think about. I managed to lower the rail at the head of my bed. Then, while lying flat, I turned to the foot of the bed. I threw the pillowcase off the bed. I fell to the floor with my hands down first and my feet and legs still on the bed. As I fell, I noticed my IV pole. If I could take it with me, I would live longer. As I reached for it I knocked my Bible open, but I didn't want to see what it said. I was weak, sick, crying, and just wanting to be free for a little while. I couldn't see well, and I couldn't breathe well. I kept telling myself, "You can make it outside and to the woods next door." I lay flat on the floor, closed my eyes, and prayed.

"Dear Lord, you know my heart and how I long to be physically well. I need to be with my husband

and children. I need medical attention. I need to be able to drink, and I am dehydrated. Lord, help me get out of this place. Anything is possible with you. Lord, if I go outside I will possibly not live long, but if I stay here I might not live long. Lord, help me. Show me what to do. I am so weak! In Jesus' name, Amen!

I opened my eyes, and right in front of me was a banner the Girls in Action made for me. It said, "Be still and know that I am God. Psalm 46:10." They had made it huge with mountains on it. There it was: "Be still and know that I am God." It didn't say, "Be crawling, or sitting, or walking." It said, "Be still!"

I lay on the floor and sobbed. I knew not to go outside, but how could I stay in the nursing home even another day? I prayed to the Lord that whatever he had planned for me I would do. If it was to be bedridden and living in a nursing home, I would do it. As long as it glorified him and his will for my life, then so be it.

I then had to try and get back onto the bed. I put my legs up first then rolled onto the bed. That was the most desperate night of my life, but my favorite Bible verse saved me. I just had to be still and listen to God. I knew then that everything would work out in God's plan. And God did have a mighty plan for me in his time.

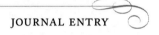

JOURNAL ENTRY

Dear Lord,

I just want to be free. I need to leave this room and this bed. I feel like I am in jail, but even people in jail get to leave their cell. Lord, please heal me. I am begging you, and I know if I believe and ask for it in Jesus' name it will happen. I want to stand next to my children and see how they have grown. I feel so trapped today; help me, Lord, as I call to you.

From Nursing Home to Hospital

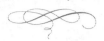

I was getting sicker and sicker. Dr. Davis came to see me on August 18, 1999. He took one look at me and said, "I am going to have to put you in the hospital. You are dehydrated; we need to see if you are sick due to the medication or because of your stomach." He gave immediate orders to start an IV and transport me by ambulance to the hospital. I was so relieved. God had heard my cry for help, and I hadn't done something stupid. I had waited on God.

Being in the hospital was to me like staying at the Holiday Inn. At least I knew there that they would take care of me physically. Thank you, Lord! Then Dr. Davis called in a gastrologist. He ran a few tests, and it was determined that I had a hernia and acid reflux disease. The high doses of beta blockers were making me sicker. I was depressed and worried, and so was Dr. Davis because he was taking me off the drug that was our only hope at the time.

All I could think about was not going back to the nursing home. I begged Dr. Davis to keep me in the hospital, please not to send me back to the nursing home. He said, "I can't let you stay here." After five days of harsh IVs and a new medication for my stomach, I began to eat and drink. The food was good and hot. The nurses were extremely nice and took good care of me. It really makes a difference when they really care.

My son's birthday was August 22. My friend Nancy made a cake, and we had a party at the hospital for him. I couldn't help but wish that I would be able to give him a real mom as a birthday present, a mom who could be home with him, who could take care of him.

Fear rushed all through my body every time I thought of having to go back to the nursing home. I begged the doctor and everyone not to send me back. My doctor decided to try me on another type of drug and overdose me on it. Proamatine was the drug I used in the study with Dr. Cecil Coughlin to increase my blood pressure. So he began overdosing me on Proamatine. With Dr. Davis trusting in medicine and me trusting in God, we carried on.

The next day I woke up, and the first thing I did was look at my body. I actually felt good. I had a blood pressure. Wow! I was no longer on a roller coaster. I could breathe, and my chest wasn't pounding. It was a good feeling I had never felt before. It didn't seem like my body. The doctor came in and said, "Hey, we're onto something. You actually have a registered blood pressure. I think I'll keep you a couple more days. " I again begged him not to send me back to the nursing home.

He said, "Let's try and sit you up!" I was all for it. It had been years since I had sat up without passing out.

The physical therapist kept saying, "Even if the drugs work to keep your blood pressure up, your muscles will be too weak for you to sit up for over several seconds at a time." Tim, the nurse, slowly raised the head of my bed. It was amazing. I didn't black out. When I did sit up, I felt human again. I felt touched by God. Everything looked wonderful because I was not looking at things from a lying-down position. It was amazing. On August 26, 1999, Tim brought a chair into my room and said, "I'll get the aides to come lift you up. Let's see if you can sit in this chair for about five minutes." He said, "Remember, don't expect much. It's been a long time since you have sat up." I told him I could get into the chair without help, and I did. I sat up for ten hours that day. The nurses and the doctor were amazed. I was amazed. How great thou art, Lord. How great thou art. "Thank you, Lord," was all I could say.

The next day they decided to put me into a wheelchair. They did, and I wheeled up and down the halls, in and out of rooms. I actually took a shower by myself, the first one in years. I got in the shower, and

I was yelling, "Oh, this feels great! Oh man, this feels wonderful! Oh, this is awesome!" I yelled so loud that the person two doors down thought something was wrong with me. The nurse was sent to check on me and see what in the world was going on. The fourth-floor nurse and staff were amazed; they had shared my miracle with me. I went from being completely bedridden to sitting up. I dressed myself, showered, and brushed my own hair, and I did it all by myself. That felt wonderful.

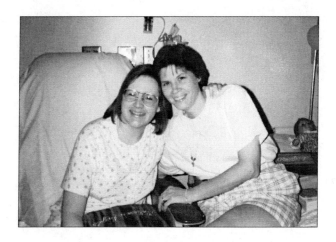

I finally heard the words I had prayed for. Dr. Davis said, "We will not send you back to the nursing home; you can eventually go home after we keep an eye on your medication for a few more days." God answered my prayer in his time. He sent me the doctor I had prayed for. God showed me just to be still and know that he is God.

Dear Lord,

I am so excited! I can go home! Wow! You have answered my prayers in your time. I was also able to take a shower. It felt wonderful, marvelous! Thank you, Lord, for answering my prayers and the prayers of so many on my behalf. I am humbled. Words cannot express how excited I feel to be touched by you, my Lord and Savior. I praise your name.

Dear Lord,

I have to thank you again. Thank you for helping me be able to go home. I feel that if I write it over and over I will eventually believe it. I get to go home.

My Finest Hour

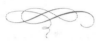

After I had sat up ten hours in a chair we decided to try and have me stand. I was told not to expect anything since it had been years since I had stood up or walked. I went down to the physical therapy room and stood. I only lasted forty seconds. Every day we kept trying, but it seemed hopeless. I could only last forty seconds, but I wouldn't give up.

The head nurse, Brenda, and the therapist took me downstairs to try to walk one more time. I stood up while holding onto the parallel bars and put one foot in front of the other, then again. I walked! They checked my blood pressure, and I was *walking* with a good blood pressure. I walked all around the room. I fell to my knees, sobbing with joy. The physical therapist looked shocked because all of his training had taught him that people get weak if they lie in bed too long. But there I was, bedridden for years and walking. I was so humbled. The feeling of God's mighty touch was amazing, for God heard my cry for help. I will never forget the feeling of joy I had the day God touched my life. "You are my lamp, O Lord; the Lord turns my darkness into light. With your help I can advance against a troop; with my God I can scale a wall" (2 Samuel 22:29–30, NIV). God took me from the dark nursing home to light. I am so thankful I didn't escape that desperate night at the nursing home. I waited on God, and he rescued me.

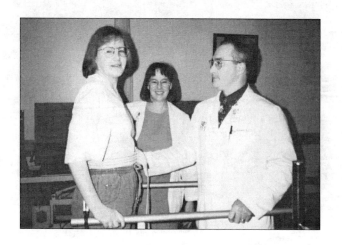

As for God, his way is perfect, the word of the Lord is flawless. He is a shield for all who take refuge in him. For who is God besides the Lord? And who is the Rock except our God. It is God who arms me with strength and makes my way perfect.

2 Samuel 22:31–33, NIV

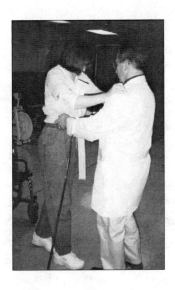

The head nurse asked if I wanted to walk into the elevator and to my own room. I said yes. When the elevator doors opened up, all the staff saw God's miracle. They all started clapping and crying. I was sobbing at what God and Dr. Davis had done for me, and so were the nurses and aides. They cried, and I hugged each and every one of them. There is nothing like feeling God's spirit when he touches your life. It can't compare to anything. I couldn't sit down. Even though they kept telling me to take it easy, I couldn't.

I called my pastor and told him I was walking. He went running through the church saying, "Lynn is walking!" As he ran through the church praising God and telling everyone I could walk, he entered the choir room, and the senior adult choir was practicing the "Hallelujah Chorus." When they heard the news, they started singing with even greater praise.

Soon he came to see for himself. As he stood at the door I walked to him, and we sobbed.

Then I called a dear friend who had always been there for me. He came to the door, and I walked to him. I surprised my husband; I walked to him and gave him a really big hug. People who had prayed years for me to walk flooded the hospital to see the miracle for themselves. It was glorious! What a joy to have prayers answered! I was so glad I hadn't given up.

Now I wanted to surprise my sweet children who hadn't seen their mom walk in years. I was sitting in a wheelchair at the end of the hall. When they got off the elevator I ran to them. Tricia screamed,"Momma, Momma!" Kenneth was smiling from ear to ear. What a glorious day we had. What a miracle God had performed. My sweet children would finally have their mother home with them again. While standing in the hospital hall, we cried and laughed with happiness at the joy that I could not only sit up, but I could also walk. My son asked me, "Does this mean you can make me your homemade spaghetti?"

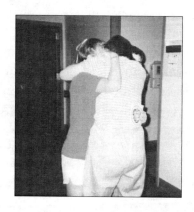

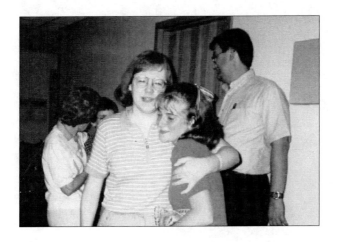

My daughter said, "What about your mashed potatoes?"

Then my son said, "Mom, I know it is good and all, but who is going to share Jesus with the people in the nursing home if you aren't there?"

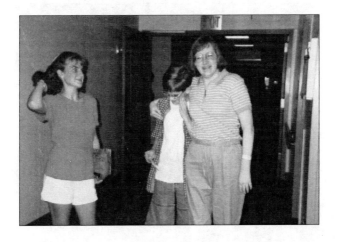

Nothing is impossible with God.

Luke 1:37, NIV

He gives strength to the weary and increases the power of the weak.

Isaiah 40:29, NIV

Trust in him at all times, O people; pour out your hearts to him, for God is our refuge.

Psalm 62:8, NIV

Come near to God and he will come near to you. "Come to me, all you who are weary and burdened, and I will give you rest."

Matthew 11:28, NIV

The Lord is my strength and my shield; my heart trusts in him, and I am helped. My heart leaps for joy and I will give thanks to him in song.

Psalm 28:7, NIV

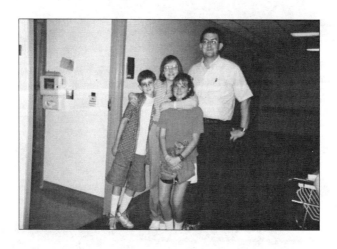

When no one heard my cry, when no one could help me, God did. He came when my heart trusted in him alone. My hospital room was on the fourth floor, and I could see the nursing home from my window. I thanked God I didn't have to go back there. I thanked God for saving me; he had heard my cry and come to my rescue.

Dr. Davis came in and asked me if I was brave, and I said I was. He said, "Then you can go home on the fourth of September." I stood up and walked to him. He had never seen me up. He said I was tall, and I told him he was smart.

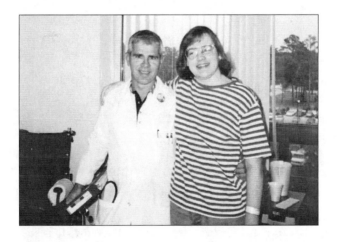

On September 3, 1999, I woke up and felt like I had dreamed it all. I got up at two a.m. and walked all over the room then went back to bed. The next day the therapist walked me around the halls, one thousand square feet. I walked so much the therapist was out of breath, and I wasn't.

I didn't own clothes or shoes since I had been in the bed for so long. A friend of mine bought me some clothes; another bought me some makeup and a curling iron; still another bought me my first pair of shoes. The next day I would go home.

JOURNAL ENTRY

Dear Lord,

You heard my cry. I sat up for ten long hours. I could feel your arms holding me up. I can feel your mighty touch. I will never be the same. Then I actually walked. It was so awesome surprising my children when they got off the elevator. Their smiles, along with Ken's, were a vision I will never forget. Thank you, Lord, for everything. Thank you for Jesus Christ. Thank you for Dr. Davis and his staff. Wow!

JOURNAL ENTRY

Dear Lord,

I can hardly believe it. I can walk. Wow! It is so awesome to be able to put one foot in front of the other and walk. I can't thank you enough, for you are mighty, and I know it. When no one could help me, you did. That just proves I should rely on you instead of people. I understand that now, God. Thank you.

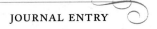

JOURNAL ENTRY

Dear Lord,

Just think, I can stand up by the window and see outside. The sky is beautiful. The trees look fantastic. I can see cars zooming by. I can't wait to ride in a car. That will be so cool. Thank you, Lord, for helping me use the restroom alone, brush my teeth alone, and wash my hair alone. It feels wonderful!

God Touched My Life

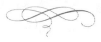

I couldn't sleep. All I could think about was going home for the first time in a year. September 4, 1999, was the day I would get to ride in our car for the first time and walk into my house for the first time. I am so thankful to God for rescuing me. "I will praise the Lord all my life; I will sing praise to my God as long as I live" (Psalm 146:2, NIV).

The Opelika/Auburn News would be at my house for an interview. I was going home with my husband at ten a.m. to be with my family! Ken pulled the car up. It felt funny to sit up in a car. He drove off, and we waved goodbye and drove down the road. Everything had changed. I couldn't even tell you how to get to my house. I had only been in and out of my house by ambulance.

As we pulled up, I was touched to see so many people there to greet me. They had balloons and smiles on their faces at the miracle they were watching. As I opened my car door, I was so overwhelmed. I had to put my head down. I cried with joy. I told the crowd that, through their prayers and support, God had helped me to walk. I walked through my yard and stopped and looked out into the crowd. There were so many friends who had been faithful for years. I praised God's holy name for all of them.

I told the crowd, "Thank you for all your prayers." I stopped and saw Kenneth in the crowd and grabbed him and Tricia. I was at home. I walked through the yard and up the gravel to my house. I looked down at my feet, and they were actually stepping forward through the gravel. I hadn't tried stairs yet. I said, "Here I go." It was no problem. I walked into my house for the first time ever! I felt like a giant because for the past five years I had only seen people from a lying-down position. What a true blessing!

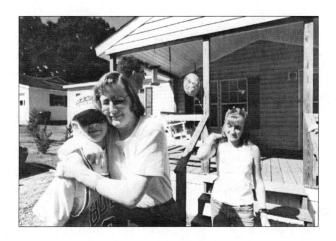

I was home at last. I jumped right into cooking, cleaning, and taking care of my family. I made Kenneth his homemade spaghetti. He was so happy to have Mom's cooking that he licked the pot. We all sat at the table, held hands, and prayed. What a blessing to have answered prayers. The smile on Kenneth's face as he ate my spaghetti was a vision I will always remember. I was finally able to take care of my family.

The things I had missed the most were eating together and tucking my kids into bed at night and praying together. I had missed all the ballet recitals, band performances, and baseball games. I was finally home. For months I had tears in my eyes. I was able to do things, things I was grateful for like cleaning the bathroom. I never dreamed cleaning would be a dream come true.

The world had changed so much while I had been bedridden. The speed limit was higher. Money looked different. Even the phone seemed to ring faster. All of a sudden, I didn't fit in the world. It had changed so much, but that was okay because the Bible speaks about not being of the world. I was glad Jesus Christ was still the same because that is where my hope is.

For the next week I worked in the house, and I was very emotional about just being home. The only time I rested was when I studied God's Word. Every day I opened the front door and yelled out into the yard, "Joy comes in the morning!" and "God is so good!" The mailman was putting mail in our box, and I had yelled out the door that God is so good.

He said, "I guess so." I told him I knew so and shared my testimony with him. I hope God planted a seed into his heart so he will one day find Jesus.

A week after being home I started studying Peter and Paul in prison and how prison then was bad compared to today. In the journal I had in the nursing home, I had written how much I would rather be in jail instead of the nursing home. After all, in jail you can get your teeth cleaned, have your hair cut, and have three hot meals a day. Plus, you can have medical help at any time. It sounded good to me while I was living in the nursing home.

While I was reading my Bible about Paul in prison the phone rang. I answered it, and a man asked to speak to Lynn Adams. He said, "I will have to send a sheriff to pick you up. You owe the ambulance company four hundred dollars. Can you pay it today?" I told him I had had no idea that I owed that money and that I had just gotten home from an extended stay in a nursing home. I asked him not to take me to jail. The sheriff did come, and Ken and I paid him the money. Thank goodness I was not sent to jail. I knew from then on to be careful what I prayed for.

JOURNAL ENTRY

Dear Lord,

I can't wait to ride in our car for the first time. I can't wait to see how to get to my house. I can't wait to be home with my family. I have longed for this day for a year. Thank you, God, for touching my life. I can never repay you for the things you have done for me. I love you, Lord. I will always share what you have done for me in my life, whether sick or well.

JOURNAL ENTRY

Dear Lord,

Today I cleaned the bathroom. It was so much fun. I put on a load of clothes, and it was fun. I can't believe I can do all these things. Thank you so much. I will keep praising your name. Oh, I actually made my kids their lunch. Wow! That is a first! They enjoyed not having to do it themselves.

First Day at Church

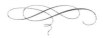

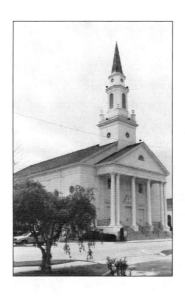

On Sunday, September 19, 1999, I rode to church with
my family and walked into the First Baptist Church
of Opelika. What another miracle! It felt wonderful
to be in God's house with God's people. I had tears
in my eyes and chill bumps on my arms. I could most

definitely feel the presence of our Lord. For years I had prayed to be able to sit with my family in church. I was so overjoyed to be in God's house that I immediately started sobbing. While the church was beautiful, the people who were there made it God's house.

I couldn't believe I was finally there. It was so much better than having church in the nursing home alone. I looked around and saw all the caring people who had continued to pray, bring meals, and support me. It was a true blessing to be able to attend church.

When we sang I sobbed. When we prayed I sobbed. Everything was heavenly, a dream that had come true, It could only be a miracle. What a blessing. I cried as I looked at my young son and teenage daughter sitting beside me. That is what family is all about in God's eyes, sitting together and worshiping together. My children had grown up so much. I had missed so many events in their lives, but I tried not to focus on that. I would have to put that in the past and celebrate now.

Brother Ron spoke on Psalm 73:23–26.

> Yet I am always with you; you hold me by my right hand. You guide me with your counsel, and afterwards you will take me into glory. Whom have I in heaven but you? And earth has nothing I desire besides you. My flesh and my heart may fail, but God is the strength of my heart and my portion forever.

It was the same scripture I had read at the hospital when I first walked. The scripture talks about the earth having nothing. But there I was, finally in the world. I sure didn't feel like I was a part of the world, and I prayed I would never be of the world, just of God. The last part of the scripture says God is my strength, and I had certainly lived those words. "I can do anything through him who gives me strength" (Philippians 4:13, NIV). With God you can do anything, I learned that again on that glorious day when I attended church.

I looked around into the crowd, and some people didn't look happy to be in church. It was like they were robots having to go. All I could think about was what a blessing and how awesome it was for me. People do not realize how blessed they are. I kept saying "Amen," and my daughter told me they didn't do that anymore. Indeed, the world had changed. I cried all through the service, resulting with a pile of tissues on the floor. When I say a *pile,* I mean several inches high.

At the end of the service, during the prayer, I walked down the aisle of the church. I wanted to join in person because more than a year before, I had written a letter saying I wanted to join the church. I had told people that one day I would walk into church, and I knew it would happen in God's time. I waited on the Lord.

"Wait for the Lord; be strong and take heart and wait for the Lord" (Psalm 27:14, NIV).

"I wait for the Lord, my soul waits, and in his word I put my hope" (Psalm 130:5, NIV).

I had trusted and waited on the Lord, and in his time, he helped me attend church.

The pastor at first did not want me to speak. I

had called him at home and asked if I could share at church what God had done in my life. He didn't share the pulpit much. I asked him, "How would you feel if you had prayed for years and years to be able to attend church? Wouldn't you want to share God's miracle?" I told him God wanted me to speak. So during the closing prayer, I walked down the aisle and experienced the miracle God had performed. I walked all the way down to the front. It was so humbling. As I looked out into the crowd, I could see so many faces of people who loved me and had helped me through all those years. I was so touched. As I began to share my testimony, all the pain went away. God spoke through me. I used to be so shy and afraid to speak, but God had touched my life. When God touches your life, it is not a *maybe* that you share your testimony but a *must*.

The pastor handed me the microphone. I explained how exactly one month ago I had been living in a nursing home, flat on my back, unable to sit up. No one could help me, but God did. He heard my cry. Yes, my doctor can take credit for helping my blood pressure, but only God can help someone walk all alone without being dizzy after being bedridden for five years. That wasn't medically possible, but with God it certainly was possible.

I talked about how money looked different and that even getting gas for my car was different. The speed limit was higher. Things had changed so much. But I shared how "Jesus Christ is the same yesterday, today, and forever" (Hebrews 13:8). I shared how it is never too late to accept Jesus Christ into your heart.

He is still waiting on people to accept him. I am so thankful that Jesus Christ is the same so that others can become saved. He never changes.

God showed people that day in church who didn't believe in miracles that miracles still happen. I shared how everyone is blessed to be able to get up and attend church. The important things to me are spending time praying with my family, eating together, and attending church together. I shared that with God, nothing is impossible.

As I looked around, I saw tears streaming down so many faces. My church family was witnessing a miracle.

"Have faith in God," Jesus answered. "I tell you the truth, if anyone says to this mountain, 'Go, throw yourself into the sea,' and does not doubt in his heart but believes that what he says will happen, it will be done for him."

Mark 11:22–23, NIV

Consider it pure joy, my brothers, whenever you face trials of many kinds, because you know that the testing of your faith develops perseverance. Perseverance must finish its work so that you may be mature and complete, not lacking in anything.

James 1:1–4, NIV

I waited patiently for the Lord; he turned to me and heard my cry. He lifted me out of the slimy pit, out of the mud and mire; he set my feet on a rock. And gave me a firm place to stand.

Psalm 40:1–2, NIV

As I was speaking that day at church I was so calm and filled with love because when God lays something on my heart to share, I do not get nervous. I simply speak. This is a miracle because as a child and teenager, I was afraid to speak to people. I would get nervous. That Sunday, God spoke through me and revealed his glory. Brother Ron ended up asking me to come back and share my story with the eleven o'clock service and, of course, I said I would. It felt so good and joyous to share God's miracle. At the eleven o'clock service I wasn't done speaking when Brother Ron tried to take the microphone away from me, and I ran. Everyone laughed. I just wasn't finished sharing what God had done in my life.

Words cannot express the feeling of joy and peace I had that day in church. The love of my church family was so great, and I was so blessed to have them all as a part of my life.

JOURNAL ENTRY

Dear Lord,

I can't believe it. I was in church. With your miracle I was able to walk down and join the church in person and share how you have blessed me. It was wonderful, and I will always thank you for that day. Your love is mighty. I was touched as I looked around the church and saw so many people sobbing. Most of them had been praying along with me. What a blessing.

Two Amazing Trips

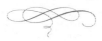

Ken had a business trip to take to the Grand Ole Opry Hotel. It was October, and I had only been home from the nursing home for a month. I decided to go along with him. After all, I was free from my bedroom, nursing home, and house. While Ken was driving there I kept saying, "Wow! Look at that tree! Wow! Look at the sky! Wow! Look at that bird!" I had never fully appreciated God's beauty. It was so exciting.

We arrived at the hotel, and it was all so beautiful. The hotel had such lush greenery and flowers everywhere, with a stream that ran through it. While Ken was in his first meeting I went outside, lifted up my hands toward heaven, and said, "Thank you, Lord." I was physically and spiritually free. Ken and I even went out to eat one night. Being out with my husband was also a miracle that came true; it had been years. What we ate didn't matter; it could have been peanut butter and jelly. We were just happy to be sitting at a table across from each other.

I didn't have clothes for the trip because I had spent the previous several years in pajamas. One of the Sunday school classes at my church bought me an outfit. I was dressed and walking up and down the halls at the hotel. I have to admit it was a little scary. But I can't describe how good it was to be free. While Ken was in classes I found so many pretty places inside and outside to study my Bible. I saw flowers, trees, waterfalls—all of God's beauty. I thanked God for the opportunity to get out of town. God is so very good to me.

After being home for several months I began to try and find a Christian radio station to listen to. I still did not fit in the world. God had touched my life, and I would never be the same. I couldn't stand television; I wanted to hear some gospel music. I found a radio station called The Well. They had almost no advertising and played music about Jesus. It was uplifting in this world of sin and violence to hear songs about God. I felt burdened to call them and share God's miracle and how he had touched my life. I began to listen for a location or phone number. For days, they never said.

I called information and told them the name and where their listening areas were. The operator said there was no such radio station. My friends and my husband said, "Just forget it. What's the big deal?" But I was still burdened and unable to sleep. I found myself praying for the radio station while I listened to it. I felt very strongly about God wanting me to talk to someone at the station. I asked people if they had ever heard of The Well. They had, but no one knew where it was. Two weeks later I called the number an operator gave me. When a girl answered the phone, she said, "The Well." I immediately started sharing what God had done in my life. I was so excited that I didn't give her a chance to talk. When I was finished talking, she said, "Ma'am, this is a gas station … But you know, after what you have shared with me, I just might start believing in God." I shared Jesus with a young lady working in a gas station in Fairhope, Alabama.

After this I was burdened even more to find the radio station. Ken said, "Lynn, I'll call the First Baptist Church of Horseshoe Ben. They just had an advertisement for them. They will know."

Ken called and talked with the secretary, who said, "Yes, I know the radio station. They changed their name awhile back. I can give you the number." Finally I had a number.

I began to pray for God to give me the right words to say. I wasn't sure why the Lord wanted me to contact them. After I prayed, I called, and a lady answered. I said, "Is this the radio station The Well?" She said it was, and I began to share with her what had happened in my life.

She began to cry! She said, "You are an answer to our prayers. Our radio station is having financial difficulty, and we are fixing to give up, shut down."

I said, "If you give up today, tomorrow might

be the day the Lord answers your prayers." I shared some scripture with her on prayer while she cried.

She said, "It is good to know people are listening to our radio station. My husband and I own it. We attend the Lake Martin Baptist Church." I reminded her how the devil would love for the radio station to close down because it glorifies God. She said, "You're right." I told her the devil tried his best to hinder me from finding her phone number, but I hadn't given up.

She later called me back, saying the Lord laid it on her heart for me to speak on the radio station. My friend Brenda set out with me to the radio station. When we arrived we were greeted with hugs and put in a room so we could talk on the radio. I shared my testimony on the air. Then I talked about how the radio station was in trouble, and I said we needed to "fill the well." I told people to please give what they could so the radio station could stay open.

The radio station was the last place I went before passing out again. Although I am thankful for those six months, it was difficult when my condition worsened again. It felt like my life was quickly snatched away. I could feel my body working against me; no matter how hard I tried, I was getting sicker. I started passing out almost daily. I cried and pleaded with God to help me. Ken and my children were heartbroken.

Back then I couldn't understand why the Lord allowed me to become so ill again. Dr. Davis said my body got used to the medication, and it just didn't work on me anymore. Since I was already overdosed on it, we couldn't up the medication any more.

Years later I could understand why it happened,

for God has used my life in so many ways I never dreamed possible. If I had stayed well, would I have been too busy to help others with my condition? Probably so. Although I wanted to return to work and drive, I was never able to do that. The one thing I could do was pray. Being homebound and bedridden gave me hours to pray, not only for my family, but also for others who suffer from dysautonomia.

Only the Lord knows how many people I have talked to and comforted with the same love Jesus had given me. Even though I was taken out of the world again physically, I still had my spirit, and it was strong, thanks to the Lord.

The next two years, I really struggled with constant infections and surgeries.

Once, when I was in the hospital, an employee named Alma told me that she had bad days but that she listened to a radio station called The Well. She told me how much it helped her after her husband died.

JOURNAL ENTRY

Dear Lord,

I am glad The Well is still up and running. I will never forget talking on it and sharing what you have done in my life. Thank you for the opportunity.

I am slipping back into bad health. I do not know what to do. I am heartbroken because I have had a taste of being free. Now, after six months, I am bedridden again. Lord, you know my needs and what is best for me. Follow through with your plans, whether I am sick or well. Use me in any way you would like to. Even though I am upset about not being able to walk again, I still love you with all my heart. I know in my grief you will supply me with your peace, joy, and love.

JOURNAL ENTRY

Dear Lord,

I want so much to be well. I feel really bad. I am so sick I can hardly stand it. Please comfort me once again. Take me in your arms and shower me with your love. I need you.

JOURNAL ENTRY

Dear Lord,

Thank you for allowing me to walk for six months. It was so joyous. I am torn apart because I am again unable to walk without passing out. If I never walk again, I know I will walk when I get to heaven, and I will no longer suffer because Jesus came into the world to save me.

The Lion's Club

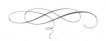

In June of 2001 I contacted the Opelika Lion's Club because The National Dysautonomia Research Foundation (NDRF) was in danger of closing down. Although my own family was struggling financially, I felt that the dysautonomia patients needed help more than my family did. God does want us here on earth to help others. I couldn't let NDRF close because it is the only foundation where people who suffer from dysautonomia can get support and be educated on the different types of the condition. We needed money to print booklets and educate doctors on the condition, and of course, people needed support to get through the rough days of living with dysautonomia.

I got to work on the Internet and asked people who suffer from dysautonomia to write to the Opelika Lion's Club and tell them how the condition had impacted their lives. The Lion's club received desperate letters from everywhere begging for help. The Lion's Club is an organization that usually only helps the blind. Dysautonomia patients do not have an organization to help them. It was important that dysautonoima patients share with the Lion's Club about their everyday struggles of trying to live with dysautonomia.

After reading all the letters, they agreed to help us. The Lion's Club sold mops, brooms, and other things and raised six thousand dollars. What a blessing it was to be able to keep the foundation up and running. If it had not been for the Lion's Club's help, the NDRF would have had to close down. Then no one would be able to get support.

The foundation is run by Christian people who really care for others. The CEF of the NDRF years ago found out she had a type of dysautonomia. At that time she asked her physician where she could find a support group or a place where she could get information. The doctor said, "There is no such place." That is when she decided, along with God, to start a foundation for herself and others. Throughout the years, the foundation has grown. We still need support so we can keep helping others and print pamphlets to educate people and doctors on the condition.

I admire and thank God for Linda and Dan Smith and the sacrifices they have made to keep the foundation alive and growing. They do not get paid for all their hard work. We still need your help. If you would like to donate, the website is www.ndrf.org. Thank you, Lord, and continue to use the foundation to help and educate others. One day the word *dysautonomia* will be a word accepted like the word *cancer* is today. Someone was a pioneer for cancer research, and Linda and Dan Smith are pioneers for dysautonomia. Thank you, Opelika Lion's Club, for all your hard work and all your help. You cannot even fathom how much you have helped numerous people.

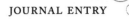

JOURNAL ENTRY

Thank you, Lord, for the Lion's Club and the generous donation they have given to the National Dysautonomia Research Foundation. It will help so many people. I will still be able to support others in their time of need through the NDRF. I love the people of the Lion's Club, for they heard my cry for help.

Levophed

Dr. Davis was at a seminar in July of 2001 and learned some new things about a drug called Levophed. He had known about the drug but now had an idea to use it in a different way to help me sit up. His nurse called me and said, "We have a drug we can try on you that will help you sit up."

There I was getting my hopes up. What did I have to lose? The drug was so strong that in medical school, it was called *Lethalphed*. It is a drug used on people who have very low blood pressure or no blood pressure at all. It is administered to bring them back to life. Dr. Davis had a plan to administer it to me in the form of IV that would run continuously to keep my falling blood pressure up. The risk would be that when my blood pressure hit a normal rate, Levophed could make my blood pressure go too high, and that could cause a stroke. I had to do a lot of praying before I decided to try it out.

I was admitted into the intensive care unit at East Alabama Medical Center to try the drug for three months. I needed to be monitored daily. When I arrived I was given the paperwork on the drug. I felt like someone had to try it out, so why not me? I prayed for guidance from the Lord, and I trusted Dr. Davis.

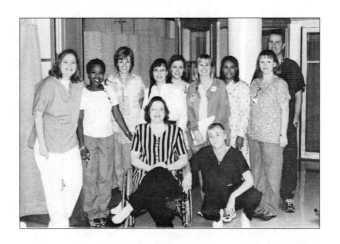

I have to admit that I was nervous when they started the drug. My heart felt like it was going to pound out of my chest. It did help me sit up in a recliner, and I actually had a blood pressure. Dr. Davis said, "Just the fact that you are responding to it means it's working." I was happy it was working; we didn't know what it would do to me long- or short-term. Dr. Davis wanted to see how the drug worked while I was living normally. He asked me where I would like to go. My daughter was entered in the

Junior Miss Pageant, and I wanted to go see her perform. Everyone in the ICU worked on getting me ready for my outing. The nurses fixed my hair, did my makeup, and brought me an outfit to wear to the occasion.

We went to the Opelika Performing Arts Center and watched my daughter perform, dance, and flow across the stage. I had tears in my eyes watching her grace and beauty. I was so proud of her inner beauty as well as her outer beauty. I was thrilled to be there.

On the way back to the hospital I passed out on the two nurses. That resulted in a man from the ICU carrying me to a stretcher. Then I was placed in my bed in the unit. Thanksgiving came while I was in the ICU. A friend of mine brought me some of the dinner she had cooked for her family, and it was delicious. The Opelika Band was marching on television in a Thanksgiving Day parade. I was screaming, "All right! Go! Yay!" as I watched my son on television play his trombone.

While I was in the hospital my daughter turned eighteen. Like many of her other birthdays, this one would be spent with me in the hospital. The staff helped me decorate my room so it didn't look like a hospital room. A friend of Tricia's called her friends to come. We surprised her. I told her how she was my Junior Miss. I had bought her a tiara, and I placed it on her head and told her how much she meant to me, how she was one of the things in my life I had done right. I told her how she had inspired me to hang in there when things were hard.

After a three-month stay in the intensive care unit, I was able to go home. I must say thank you to all of the staff for their courage and help. It was always a group effort. When I arrived home and walked into my house, I saw a new recliner. The staff from the ICU had bought it for me.

I stayed on Levophed for the next several years, even though we didn't know what it would do to me long-term. It did help me attend a few things I wanted to attend.

I was able to reach the two most important goals I had set for myself. I was able to see both of my children graduate with honors from Opelika High School, and I was able to go to Washington, DC and speak on Capitol Hill. I wouldn't have been able to do those things without Levophed.

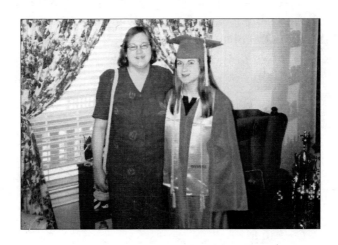

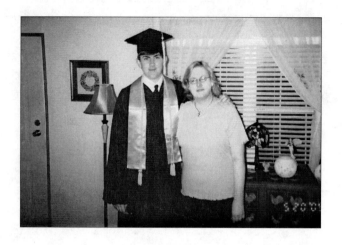

I used Levophed from 2001 until 2007; then the side effects really began to take a toll on me. Although getting off the drug meant a different physical life for me, I had no choice. The IV supplier at East Alabama Infusion Center closed, and all the other suppliers in the area said Levophed could only be used in ICU—that it was illegal to use in the home—so I no longer had access to the drug. My life again changed. Without the Levophed it would be much harder to function. I would have to spend most of my days in bed or in my recliner.

JOURNAL ENTRY

Dear Lord,

Thank you for the drug Levophed. Although we are not sure what it will do to me physically, it does allow me to go places. I went to see my children graduate from high school, and I was able to go to Washington, DC and speak on Capitol Hill. If it weren't for all the caring staff in the ICU ward, I wouldn't have gotten to do those things. Thank you, Lord, for Carolyn, Lynn, and Tim and Dr. Davis's staff. They really care and understand what I go through. Dr. Davis still amazes me because he still comes up with ways to help my blood pressure.

Lynn goes to Washington, DC

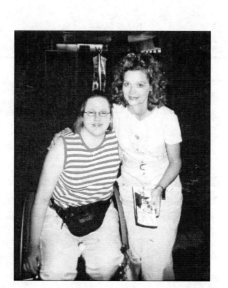

In July of 2002, Ken, Tricia, and I drove to Atlanta with Janice, a nurse and friend. From there we all flew to Washington, DC. Months earlier, I had heard that the National Dysautonomia Research Foundation was having a conference in Washington. I knew immediately I needed to speak on Capitol Hill. I called the president of NDRF and told her I wanted to speak. When she asked why, I said, "Because God wants me to." And he certainly did.

I began to call members of Congress asking them to come and listen. It was very hard to get a response. I didn't give up, I called and called, and I faxed. At the time I couldn't sit up much, so I faxed with my toes. It was challenging, but I got the job done. I sent out more than fifty faxes. No one was listening. No one responded. So I asked God to supply me with the right tools to make them hear me.

He gave me an idea. At the time, a celebrity was featured on television supplicating Congress to help with Parkinson's Disease research. He said researchers needed help and money. Since we did not have a celebrity with dysautonomia, we were ignored. But God loves us all.

I had to get the attention of Congress somehow. I decided to get people to sign my dress and jacket that I would wear to Capitol Hill. That way they would know I was important to someone. I got over one thousand signatures. I e-mailed and called the members of Congress and told them about the dress and how dysautonomia patients were important too.

After we flew in and arrived at the hotel, I couldn't wait to meet Linda. We had e-mailed and talked on the phone since 1999 but had never met in person. The NDRF is located in Minnesota. I called Senator Paul Wellstone of Minnesota and told his assistant that it was a shame he wouldn't see the NDRF group while they were in Washington. After all, it was founded in his state. They finally called Linda and told her Senator Wellstone would meet with us while we were in Washington. Senator Wellstone happened to be on the health committee. As we talked with him he said he would help us. Unfortunately, he died later in a plane crash.

I knew I would never get into the Senate building again; they were so strict, especially because it hadn't been long since 9/11. Even though I could hardly sit up, Ken and I went up and down all those long halls in the Senate building. I was determined to speak with Alabama's senator, Jeff Sessions. He was also on the health committee. We finally found his office, and I refused to leave without seeing him. I said, "I know I'm not a celebrity, but in God's eyes we are all the same. Give me a chance to speak as if I were a celebrity." I got my point across.

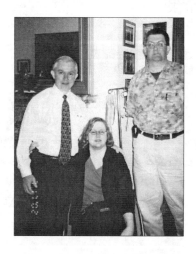

Senator Sessions happened to be on the Senate floor voting. I waited for him, and he came in and met with my husband and me. I explained the condition, how we needed help, and how one million Americans were suffering. I shared how I was the voice for so many who couldn't even leave their homes. I told him that the only reason I was there was that I was on a very strong drug. Meanwhile, the bus was waiting outside for us with everyone already on it. They ended up having to leave us, so we took a taxi back to the hotel.

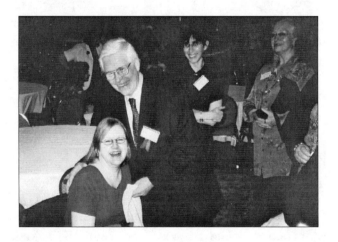

While in Washington, I spoke at the presidential dinner, where I received an award for helping the foundation by raising six thousand dollars. The best part was getting to talk to hundreds of people like me, people with all types of dysautonomia. The doctor who diagnosed me, Dr. Cecil Coughlin, was in the audience. After honoring Dr. Cecil Coughlin for his many years of work with dysautonomia patients, I talked a little about life with dysautonomia. At that time, *Survivor* was a new show on television and very popular. I told everyone that we were all "survivors." Eating worms would be easy compared to living with dysautonomia. I had everyone clapping.

I also pulled something out of my purse. A waiter thought it was a gun because it had not been long since 9/11, so he was concerned. But it was a pair of Ted hose. Linda looked at the waiter and said, "It is okay. It's just a pair of hose." Anyway, as I stood up there, I pulled those tiny hose out of my purse. They were a new pair and around six inches long and four inches wide. I told the audience, "The doctor wants me to put these on, and oh, by the way, don't get hot." If you could have seen my big body with those tiny hose held up to me you would have laughed too. With Ted hose, it takes thirty minutes to get them over your toe. If you are not someone with dysautonomia, you will not understand that, but if you are a sufferer of dysautonomia you will completely understand.

I explained how we needed a dysautonomia day, when people would give what they could to the foundation on a particular day of the year. The National Dysautonomia Research Foundation means so much to me. That is where I have met countless people who suffer from all types of dysautonomia. It has always been a blessing to help others. Most of them just wanted to know someone who understands what they are going through. I certainly understand.

There were meetings every day while I was in Washington. It was hard on my body. I would be in bed one day on an IV, and the next I would be up and speaking. One of those days, I became unconscious, but Dr. Goldstein was there to help me. The CEO of the NDRF says I risked my life to help others by finding Senator Sessions and speaking to him and by speaking to the hundreds who attended the conference. It was physically very hard to be there, but I made it with God as my strength. The conference was in 2002. From then until 2003, I was very ill. I think the trip took so much strength out of me, but it certainly was worth it, especially if it at least helped one person who was suffering.

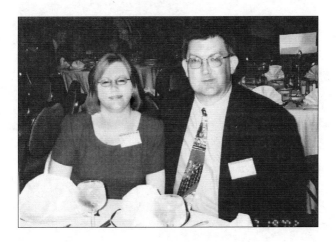

Washington is so beautiful. I feel so bad physically. I wish I could go sightseeing, but I cannot. So I will save my energy for speaking on Capitol Hill and at the president's dinner. Lord, help me say what you would want me to say. Put the words in my mouth. All the people here who have a type of dysautonomia need you. I do not know how they survive without a relationship with you.

Capitol Hill

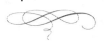

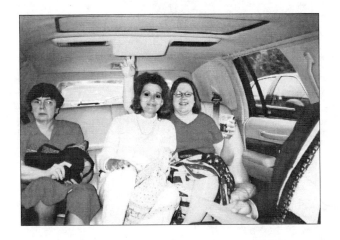

The day finally came. I would get to speak on Capitol Hill. Dr. Davis flew in for the speech and to learn more about dysautonomia from other doctors. I wore my coat, which had signatures all over it, and stated that I wasn't a celebrity but wanted to be heard. As I looked around, I noticed that the people who were there were the people I had called and faxed over and over. I was happy to see one senator in the room; the rest were employees of other members of Congress.

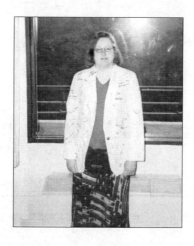

As I spoke, my doctor had tears in his eyes because of his desire just to fix me. I said, "I can see the Washington Monument from my hotel window, but I would rather be able to walk to it. I can't."

After giving the speech we headed back to the hotel in a limo. It was so good to be able to tell my story. I have always felt that God wanted me to be the voice of the million Americans who suffer from the condition.

After one more day it was time to fly home. I didn't feel very well. The plane didn't take off right away, and it was hot. I could feel myself sinking. I needed to be sitting by my husband or by Janice. The lady between Ken and me wouldn't move. She actually kept turning my air off. Ken kept telling her I had a medical condition which required me to stay cool, but she wouldn't budge. I was going to get up and move by Janice.

As soon as I stood up I passed out. My daughter and husband told me what a commotion there was on the plane. One man held the IV bag up high while other people were handing down ice, pillows, and so forth. I was unconscious. Tricia said the stewardess had to walk on the arms of the outside chairs to get by me. Once while doing so, she started to slip. Ken grabbed for her and accidentally grabbed under her skirt. It wasn't funny then, but it is now. Ken was just trying to catch her in the midst of all the commotion so she wouldn't fall. The plane landed with Janice, a doctor, and me all on the floor. An ambulance was waiting to take me off. Everyone else had to go out the back of the plane.

Although the trip made me deathly sick, I was still thankful to the Lord that I finally got to speak on dysautonomia. I hoped I had planted a seed in someone's heart. We definitely need research and acceptance in today's society. One thing I can do is pray for the people who suffer from dysautonomia.

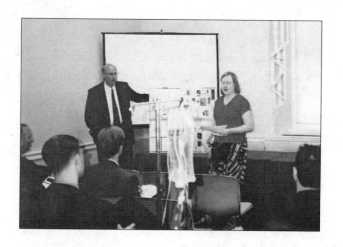

JOURNAL ENTRY

I am so blessed to be able to speak in front of people at the president's dinner with my condition. It also felt so good to speak on Capitol Hill. Even though we didn't have many there, it was wonderful to get it all out.

Capitol Hill Speech
Opening Session on Capitol Hill
July 18, 2002

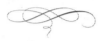

Dear Senate and Congress,

As you have already noticed I am not an actress, celebrity, or movie star. Over the last several months I have noticed quite a few celebrities addressing the Senate. I used to cry because I wanted to be heard as well. It upsets me that ordinary people do not get a chance to speak about their causes or illnesses. I have e-mailed, faxed, and called over sixty senators, congressmen, and congresswomen but have heard from only a handful. Something is wrong. But as I pondered this, I began to realize that it isn't your fault that you don't know me. So what I decided to do is have everyone who knows me and cares about me sign my dress. Please keep in mind as you listen to what I have to say that God views us all the same. Just because someone can act, or throw a ball, or has relatives in high places doesn't mean that person is more important than any of the rest of us.

There are four words I would like to address at this time. The first word is *health*. Health means the freedom from disease; it means the normal functioning of the body.

On August 4, 1994, I worked all day; then I went to my church to teach VBS. That night my life forever changed because of dysautonomia. I collapsed and was never able to get up without passing out. I can still see my son's and daughter's faces, both of which were covered with fear.

That was the last day I drove my car, the last day I walked into my place of work, and the last day I was able to stand up next to my children. For the past eight years I have been totally bedridden. My body did not function normally, and no one knew what was wrong. It took me several years to get a proper diagnosis. Because of that I lost most of my relatives. My emotional state was in trouble. Doctor after doctor turned me away, but I never gave up. In 1997 I wrote to NASA for help; after all, they are the experts when it comes to blood pressure, especially in space. After fighting and getting Senator Jeff Sessions involved, I heard from a Dr. Ralph Pelligra, who made me several suits. They helped me sit up for a few minutes, but after deflating them, I would become worse. Not long after that, I was so bad off that my family couldn't take care of me, and I was placed in a nursing home.

While in the nursing home I used a laptop. Keep in mind, I had to lie perfectly flat. I wanted to find someone else who was going through the same thing I was. That is when I found the National Dysautonomia Research Foundation. I immediately printed forty-six pages of people saying the same thing I was: "No one understands." "I can't find a doctor." "Won't someone help?" I began to e-mail everyone I could and handwrite the others.

NDRF is the only place to go for help when you suffer from an autonomic dysfunction. I am the e-mail support person and have talked with hundreds and hundreds of people who suffer. Without NDRF, they would have no help. It is time that the National Institute of Health helps NDRF support those who are suffering. We are broke and use mostly volunteers. I can't keep up with every new person I hear from. We need money to continue helping the thousands of sufferers who contact us.

The second word I want to address is *education*. In order to have good health, we need doctors who are educated on dysautonomia. It took thousands of dollars and several doctors for me to get diagnosed. The autonomic nervous system controls every aspect of the body. Why isn't there training for ANS? One million people suffer. That is more than the 882,000 people in Montana alone. That is twice as much as the 520,000 people in the Washington, DC area. What has hurt me is that most of us are not accepted, usually being turned away by uneducated doctors. When doctors aren't trained in ANS, they assume it is anxiety or depression. And when doctors don't know what is wrong with you, then husbands leave wives, thinking they have lost their minds, and family members think you are not actually ill.

The only reason I am here today is that I didn't give up, and I found a doctor who was willing to go the extra mile and do research. Dr. Davis got his education and training in the military. I think that is why he hasn't given up on me. Where most doctors would worry about getting sued, he did research to help me get out of the nursing home. We have thirty-nine doctors willing to be on our NDRF website who are trained in the ANS. Divide that by one million people, and you get 25,641 patients per doctor.

The third word I want to address is *live,* survive. On 9/11, I was bedridden, lying flat in my hospital bed. The only way I had any idea what was going on in the outside world was to listen to the news. When I saw the towers fall I felt so bad for the people in the towers because I could relate to them. After all, I had been trapped in the bed and nursing home for eight long years. *Freedom.* I felt for the world that was going to feel what I had been feeling: trapped with no choice. Our freedom as Americans was threatened. Days later, President Bush told all Americans to go about their daily lives. Well, I didn't have a life to get back to. I longed to go outside, feel the sun on my face, and see the trees. Going to the living room would have been fun.

I used to tell my friends, "Leave the door unlocked because if someone comes to rob us, maybe they will take me with them." Do you know what it is like not to be able to get your own lunch and breakfast, to lie in the bed alone at home all day, unable to go to the restroom or get a drink? There are many people in America experiencing the same thing. We want freedom to live, not the freedom only to *exist* in America, but to *live* in America. I used to be a bike rider, hiker, camper, lifeguard, employee, mother, and wife, but dysautonomia stripped me of that life.

The fourth and last word I want to address is *parent*. Especially since 9/11, it is important for children to have their parents with them. The one thing most of the women who suffer from dysautonomia have talked about is that they can't be the moms they want to be. Physically they can't cook, clean, or go to school functions. My deepest pain from dysautonomia has been losing these activities with my children. My daughter was in fourth grade when I collapsed, and my son was only six years old. I have lost eight years of their lives. I cannot get back those precious years. The day that each of my babies was born was such a special time and a gift from God. But that gift was taken away from me.

My daughter just graduated from high school. As I watched her I realized I had missed the last eight years of her life. I began to sob and had to leave the high school. Who helped her learn to ride a bike, swim, study, learn to drive? It wasn't me, and I feel so much pain from that.

My son has raised himself. He is now fourteen, and it isn't "cool" to hang out with Mom. But since he was six years old, he has dressed himself and has eaten "whatever" for breakfast. I didn't know what was going on. I was in my bed in my room, out of it, having seizures. I never got to meet his teachers or go to his school functions.

I missed eight years—96 months; 416 weeks; 2,920 days; 70,080 hours; and 4,204,810 minutes of both my children's lives.

As the e-mail support coordinator for NDRF, I have all too often listened as women shared with me that their husbands left them, that they couldn't take care of their children. That is a pain I share with numerous ladies. We just cry together. But it is time we do something to help us be the best parents we can be. Our children deserve that.

If you take the first letter in every word I have used, it spells *help*.

Health
Education
Live
Parent

·

Here is a poem written by my daughter, Tricia, when she was six years old:

Why God Made Mommies

God made Mommy to take care of her children.
God made mommies to fill the world
With love and happiness.
When something is wrong, Mommy
Is there to comfort me.
Mommies always make their
Little girls laugh and smile.
Mommies are very special, not just
On Mother's Day
But on every day.

The Ten Commandments

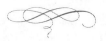

I live only forty-five minutes from Alabama's capital. In 2003 there was a controversy about whether the Ten Commandments could remain in the state judicial building. The monument was installed in the rotunda of the state judicial building in Montgomery, Alabama, on August 1, 2001. The building houses the Alabama Supreme Court. Chief Justice Roy Moore had been ordered by the 11th U.S. Circuit Court of Appeals to remove the monument because it violates the first amendment of the U.S. Constitution and its principle of separation of church and state. It was removed on August 27, 2003, and put in a storeroom that has no public access. Moore was suspended from office. He continues his fight to be reinstated and to restore the monument to the building rotunda.

This went on for weeks. It was all over the news

constantly. At the time, I was on Levophed, and it was very hot outside. One morning, I saw on the news a crowd of people in Montgomery at the state judicial building. I took one look and knew God wanted me to go.

I loaded up with ice and IVs and asked my friend Olivia if she would drive me and my sitter to the state judicial building. She said, "Only if your husband says it's okay." He said it was fine, so we all set out to go to our state capital.

When we arrived, my sitter rushed me in my wheelchair to the crowd. I stood up, walked past all of the dozens of cameramen, and went straight to the person speaking in the microphone. I said, "God wants me to speak," so he handed me the microphone.

I shared the importance of the Ten Commandments and how we need to be reminded of them. I then shared my testimony. I said, "I know there is a God because I have felt his presence." People were raising their hands and saying "Amen." I shared a brief testimony, and then it started to get hot, so I ended. One lady came up to me and said she had a brain tumor, and just by listening to what I said, she had hope in God. God took care of me that day.

Although I was on Levophed, which helped me stand, I started to get hot, and my ice bags had melted. But then it started to rain. The rain cooled things down just enough to cool me off so I could make it back to the car. What a joy it was to share God with others, especially with people who didn't believe in Jesus.

The Ten Commandments are the rules we should all live by. No one can take them away from you or me. Even though they cannot be displayed publicly, we can still study them. I suffered physically after that trip, but I knew God had wanted me to speak.

That same year, I was on Levophed. That year was so very hard; the side effects of the drug were strong. I had spells when my head would hurt so badly that I couldn't stand it. I also had spells of numbness. I would be typing away, chatting with other dysautonomia patients, and my arm would go limp; I wouldn't be able to feel it at all. My arm would actually drop by my side. It always scared me because I never knew if my feeling would come back, although Levophed did bless me by helping me to be able to be up and around more.

In 2004 I had several surgeries and infections that required a lot of hospital stays. I also had a blood clot in my jugular vein. I could still use the drug, but since it was so strong I decided I would only use it for special occasions. But I would use a Lactaid Ringer IV daily to help me. Not using Levophed caused me to be mostly bedridden again.

During 2004 I was still trying to get my parents and brother to accept my disability. But it was getting harder and harder. Every time my mother called and fussed at me to get up I got upset, which made my condition worse. My brother never listened either; my health was a subject he ignored. But I felt I couldn't give up on them. After all, they were my family, and I loved them. The pain of them not showing love to me just because I was sick was horrible.

In 2005 I still had infections, and I was in and out of the hospital. The doctors were getting concerned about the bacterial infection because it kept coming back. I focused on making scrapbooks for people. I made wedding books; birthday books; graduation books; baby books; and books of hope, love, and peace. Helping others with dysautonomia helped me through the long, lonely days.

In 2005 my mother was still talking negatively about me. One of the Ten Commandments is, "*Thou shall not bear false witness.*" I began to have prayer sessions as what to do about my parents, my brother, my sister-in-law, and my other relatives who did not accept me.

One day while I was lying in ICU, very ill, I was watching the door during visiting hours. I would look and hope to see one of my relatives walk through the door. Tears ran down my face as the time clicked on and no one came. Not only did I want them to accept me, but I couldn't travel to see them, and I missed all of them.

While I was crying, a deacon from my church entered. He asked me whom I would want our pastor to call to try and get them to understand my condition. I told him I had two aunts and a cousin I wanted to see. I waited to see the response but never heard from any of them. All of them but my cousin told my pastor he would have to speak to my mom, the one who didn't accept my illness. I still never heard from any of them.

One hot summer day in July all of a sudden I

had become very depressed. I had just had surgery the week before and was put on a new medication. I didn't feel right. So I was taken to the hospital by ambulance, where I was put in the ICU. Dr. Luscha was called in to see me. He went over my medication and said I should not be taking the new drug with my other medications because it can cause depression. So he took me off the new drug. He said he was surprised I hadn't cracked up with the two medications in my system.

Meanwhile, my husband had called my brother and told him how much I needed my family's support. So on his way home from a Baptist convention, he stopped by my house. The day my brother came I had just arrived home from the hospital. As my brother entered my room, he said, "What is wrong with you?" *Here we go again* ... I told him I had just had surgery a week before and had been put on a new drug. I also told him that the fact that my family didn't care about me was weighing heavily on my heart. It was obvious my brother did not believe me and had no sympathy. Because my brother was a minister, my relatives believed everything he said. So he had the power to go back to Florida and tell the truth, tell my relatives of my suffering, and tell them about my condition and the help I needed. But he did not. Instead he backed up what my mother kept saying, that I wasn't sick. I never thought I would lose my whole family over an illness, but it was happening.

While my brother was there that day my pastor

and his wife stopped by. I thought, *Thank you, Lord.* My pastor entered and met my brother. Then Brenda stopped by also. God sent me the support I needed. I asked my pastor to explain to my brother about my condition because he had witnessed my blacking out several times. I thought maybe since my relatives lived out of town, perhaps that was why they didn't understand, call, or come.

My brother said, "My wife said I should just put you and your junk in the truck and bring you home with me." I didn't want to be with my brother always, every day. I just wanted his love, along with his wife's, and to be accepted, but I was not. I broke down and asked him why I hadn't seen him or any of my relatives for more than a decade. They only lived three and a half hours away. My brother said it was because they were getting old. I said there had been no cards, no phone calls. I don't understand. That just wasn't true. One of my aunts who I grew up with had just gone to New York from Florida. That aunt always played the piano at church, and I always looked up to her. I thought she loved me. It had been years since I had heard from her in any way.

After we discussed all the excuses my brother made for all the relatives, I knew I had to get more stern and speak the truth.

I looked my brother in his eyes and I said, "I love you." Tears streamed down my face like a waterfall. I was waiting for my brother to tell me he loved me and that he cared about me, but he did not. I sobbed as I looked at him. My pastor's wife and Brenda were also crying. My brother told me that he couldn't support me at all because he was a minister and busy with his church. It was an obvious excuse and an ironic statement for him to make with my pastor right there in the room—my pastor, who had a membership of around four thousand while my brother had a membership of six hundred.

I said, "Have you called me over the last ten years just to see how I was?" No, he had not, but he had time to garden and oil paint and play his guitar. He just stood there and rejected me.

My pastor hugged me and said, "Well, we love this girl." That is how my pastor is; he loves people with Jesus's love. He also shows his love through actions. I told my brother I couldn't continue to carry the burden of my family's rejection, so I would let them go. I was just me, and God made me for a purpose. God made me special to be able to help and witness to others.

Brenda said, "Lynn, you need to let your family go and separate yourself from them. You cannot keep being hurt." She was crying as she said that to me because over the last decade she had witnessed the pain I had gone through trying to be accepted by my family, and that day she had witnessed my brother rejecting my plea.

Let's remember not to use the word *too busy* when it comes to your family in need. That is just an excuse. What if God said, *Sorry I'm too busy to help you today?* We would be in trouble. We should use

God as our example for the way we treat people and relatives in need.

When my brother returned to his home he called our mom and told her that I, along with my friends, had ganged up on him. I knew it was coming. My mother called, and as soon as I said hello she started yelling at me because her son was hurt. It was like he was little again and went home to tell Mommy. I hung up on my mother because she was making me upset. That was the first time I had ever done that, but there was no use in explaining anything to her because I had tried for over a decade, and she never accepted anything I said.

I pray for my brother. How can he minister and not love his own sister? I also pray for all the people who have listened to my mom over the years and haven't come to see me for themselves. "An anxious heart weighs a man down, but a kind word cheers him up" (Proverbs 12:25, NIV). For years my heart was heavy. It was like I was carrying fifty heavy bricks on my shoulders. My family never reached out to me. I was weighed down to the point that it was hurting me physically. The Bible says anyone who lets himself be distracted from the work I plan for him is not fit for the kingdom of God (Luke 9:62). So I gave all my relatives to God. Once I learned that real love comes from God, I started to feel accepted. When people from my church showed me love, it was like Band-Aids were put over the slits in my heart. Every now and then, a Band-Aid will open and pain will slip out. But it reminds me to comfort others with the comfort I have received from God and his mighty love.

> Praise be to the God and Father of our Lord Jesus Christ, the Father of compassion and the God of all comfort, who comforts us in all our troubles, so that we can comfort those in any trouble with the comfort we ourselves have received from God.
>
> 2 Corinthians 1:3–4 (NIV)

> Who shall separate us from the love of Christ? Shall trouble or hardship or persecution or famine or nakedness or danger or sword? "For your sake we face death all day long; we are considered as sheep to be slaughtered. No, in all these things we are more than conquerors through him who loved us. For I am convinced that neither death nor life, neither angels nor demons, neither the present or the future, nor any powers; neither height nor death, nor anything else in all creation, will be able to separate us from the love of God that is in Christ Jesus our Lord.
>
> Romans 8:35–39 (NIV)

Although my family greatly hurt me, I could put my hope for love in God. God showed me love, and it didn't matter that I was sick. I would no longer let my family separate me from God. I no longer had to feel that my sickness was my fault. I could just be me and what God wanted me to be, and no one could separate me from God's love.

> O God, though the mountains be shaken and the hills be removed, yet your unfailing love for me

will not be shaken not your covenant of peace be removed. You are the Lord who has compassion on me.

Isaiah 54:10 (NIV)

As the years have passed I have learned that God's love is so amazing and mighty, a love I had never felt before. I thought the pain of dealing with my family had ended. But I was wrong. I prayed for guidance from God. I would have to do the unthinkable. I had to get a restraining order against my parents because I was still being harassed by them. That day in court we agreed not to have any contact with each other. So I would not have to suffer their abuse any longer. It didn't end there; in the year 2006 I would have to face my family in court.

My Day in Court

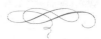

I couldn't take dealing with my parents' and brother's unbelief anymore. I am Lynn, and God made me just the way I am; he loves me. I was just wasting my energy.

One day my mom's sister came from out of town to talk with me. She hadn't seen me for a decade, so she didn't even know me. She began banging on the door. Kenneth, and I were in the living room. I saw her outside the door and knew this time I didn't have to be upset or let her in to abuse me verbally. After all, I had tried over the phone to make her understand, and she didn't. She kept banging and yelling to let her in. I ended up calling the police. As I lay on the floor of Kenneth's room with the window cracked open, I could hear her talking to the policeman. She kept saying she was there because I was insane. I know we are not supposed to worry what others think, but it was getting ridiculous. I think I saw that aunt a handful of times throughout my childhood. She had no idea who I was or what kind of person I was. I knew then that I needed the restraining order. I needed my relatives to know I wouldn't take their verbal abuse any longer.

When a person suffers from any autonomic dysfunction, stress makes the condition worse. So I had a choice to make. Would I continue to let them upset me, or would I take action so I could be the best Lynn I could possibly be? I felt so harassed and verbally abused that I could only think of one option—the restraining order against my own parents. It would be something I had to pray about for a long time. I loved my parents deeply, but I couldn't take the abuse any longer. I couldn't pretend to be well when I was not. So on March 23, 2006, we met in court. That day would be the day I lost my whole family.

My parents, brother, sister-in-law, niece, nephews, aunt, and a friend of theirs all came as if they were at war. They walked down the hall all dressed up, and they looked like they were there to win. Dr. Davis said I could only attend the hearing if I was taken by ambulance with two IVs and two paramedics. I was wheeled on a stretcher and was taken to a jury room.

There, my church family greeted me and told me that things would be okay. My church family has been there for me for twenty years. I was sad and terrified of being rejected again. But I was comforted by my eternal friends. They all knew, along with my minister, how hard I had tried to make my family believe I was sick and accept me. Tricia came running into the jury room and said, "Mom, be strong. All the relatives are here—all the ones you care about and have tried to get to come see you over the last ten years." As I began to cry Tricia said, "Mom, just tell the truth, no matter how hard it is." Not being accepted by your own family is an unimaginable pain that runs deep.

My pastor said, "Come here, everyone. Let's surround Lynn and pray for her to have the strength to get through this hearing." As I was wheeled in the courtroom I was thankful that the back of my head was toward them. I was able to speak first, in case I had to leave due to my condition.

The judge asked me what I wanted to accomplish that day. I said, "I just want my family to get some help so they will accept me. If not, I want to be left alone." He said that was very reasonable. Then I explained all the trouble they'd given me.

Little did I know, my family would get on the stand and say I was an actress, faking, and not ill. I couldn't believe it. The whole time my dad was on the stand my mom was mouthing what he should say. My lawyer asked my dad, "Do you ever want to have a relationship with your daughter ever again?"

He said, "No, not unless she is well."

That was it in a nutshell; they didn't want someone who was ill, or at least not me. Because I had to leave early due to my condition, I wasn't there for the rest of the hearing. I sobbed later when my lawyer told me the things my own brother had said about me. My brother argued about my pseudo-seizures not being real, which made the judge misunderstand my condition. I sobbed even more when I was told what my mother and father had said about me.

I had two friends testify on my behalf because they had seen me sick in the hospital. I also had Tricia and Ken speak on my behalf. My brother said my condition was not serious. My condition is severe, but even if it were mild I still would need my family to help me. He also said he had been here for my surgeries, and he had not been to a single one.

After they testified in court I knew I had to end the relationships I had with them. It was like they all died that day.

My pain was greater than any other I had ever gone through. One of the paramedics held my hand the whole time and comforted me. "So do not fear, for I am with you; do not be dismayed for I am your God. I will strengthen you and help you; I will uphold you with my righteous right hand" (Isaiah 41:10, NIV).

With a chart I explained to the judge how controlling my mom was and how she was controlling all the relatives by telling them I was not sick but insane. My lawyer began to ask me questions about my childhood and how my illness had been ignored, even back then. My mother wanted a perfect daughter, and I was not perfect.

My mom's lawyer asked me questions. He showed me a scrapbook I had made my mother. He said, "Does this look like an abusive family?"

I said, "It looks like a daughter trying to get her parents to love her." He also showed two cards I had made my mom and dad. To me, it just showed my love. I really didn't understand why my mother, father, and brother didn't accept and love me. But I knew, for my physical and emotional health, I had to let them go.

As my dad took the stand, my brother threw his Kleenex up in the air and put his hands on his head like he was crying. When it was my brother's turn to be on the stand, my lawyer asked him, "Why were you so upset about your dad? Wasn't your own sister just here on a stretcher? You didn't cry for her."

Then Ken, Tricia, and my church family took the stand in my defense. They showed they loved me and accepted me just the way I was. Patty said, "Your relatives do not know how to love you."

My daughter said, "Mom, your brother told lies while he was on the stand."

Another person who took the stand in my defense explained how my mom had threatened him one night when he came over to try and help Ken and me explain my condition to her.

Court resulted in no one winning. My mother had to pay her lawyer, and both parties agreed not to have anything to do with one another. It was a sad day. I was so hoping that my parents, brother, and other relatives would learn the truth—that I was sick, not insane or acting. The judge said it was the saddest case he had ever judged. That day I buried my blood kin. Although it was hard, I could go on and live for God and not be hindered.

Even though my parents do not want me, God does. "I am your creator. You were in my care even before you were born" (Isaiah 44:2, NIV). There it is; I am here for God, not for my parents or relatives. God cared for me and knew his plans for my life. That day in court was the last day I would allow myself to be hurt by my family. But the pain will always be a part of my heart.

Since God is love, the most important lesson is how to love. It is in loving that we are most like him. Love is the foundation of every command he has given us. The whole law can be summed up in this one command: to love each other as we love ourselves (Mark 12:31). The more time you give to something, the more you reveal its importance and value to you. The greatest gift you can give someone is your time. Words alone are worthless. "Faith by itself, if it is not accompanied by action, is dead" (James 2:17).

JOURNAL ENTRY

Dear Lord,

Help my family who have deserted me learn how to love with your love. Help me to weep for their relationships no longer. There is nothing I can do to change things. Only you can do that. I am so thankful for the many people who were in the courtroom on my behalf. They have been with me through the last decade, and they still love me. That is because they have the love of God in their hearts. I pray my family will know that even though they do not want me, I still love them. I am certainly sure that you, Lord, love me deeply. Thank you for my church family, who have helped me get through such a difficult day.

Amen.

My True Love

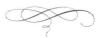

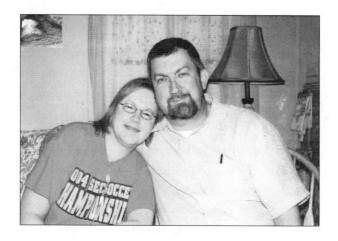

Let me tell you about a true love. Most people think of or dream about finding their one true love. When you have God's love and the person you meet also has God's love, it is for God's glory, thus giving you peace and joy, even in the midst of an illness. Our world, television, radio, and the Internet all describe true love as mostly sexual, where the women have to be thin and beautiful on the outside. As for the man, he should be muscular, tall, and make a lot of money. Most people are disappointed after marriage. Where is the love? Looks fade. Money is lost. There is no foundation to fall upon.

Who would have ever thought Ken and I would be married? As I arrived at Mobile College, a guy named Ken carried my heavy stereo into my room. That was the first time we saw each other. While I attended college, there was a live nativity scene every year. In 1981 Ken was the Joseph, and I was the Mary. As we stood there for hours on end, we would look at each other. Who would have ever thought we would eventually marry and have a son of our own.

Ken and I married young and grew up together; it has been love from the beginning. We didn't own much. We slept on a pullout couch and ate at our coffee table. We had a car that broke down every week. The odds always seemed to be against us. But we always stayed together and loved one another through all the hard times.

My husband has always worked hard at his jobs, but when I lost my job due to dysautonomia, he took on another job. Sometimes he had three jobs. While I was searching for a doctor to help me, Ken was always there. Ken always believed in me, even when my own parents did not.

We have beaten all of the odds. We have been

married for twenty-six years, and our marriage is stronger even today. We have cried together and laughed together. Ken's love is never quitting, never hating, and never ending. Ken and I have not had it easy, but through the hard times we have developed a true love through God. Ken accepts me as Lynn, just the way I am.

No, it isn't what he would want. He would rather have a healthy wife. At most weddings the minister says, "Through good and bad," and we have had it bad. "Through richer or poorer," and with high medical bills, we are poorer. "And through sickness and health," and we have lived through sickness. Three for three, and Ken has never stopped loving me.

Often, if one parent is disabled or ill, the spouse has to take on the responsibilities of the other parent. Ken always took the kids to school the first day to meet the teacher. He was always involved in their activities, like band and ballet. He drove them everywhere and taught them how to drive. Most importantly, he took them to church. While I was lying in bed, I prayed for them spiritually and found ways to help them learn about God.

> Love is patient, love is kind. It does not envy, it does not boast, it is not proud. It is not rude, it is not self-seeking, it is not easily angered, and it keeps no records of wrongs. Love does not delight in evil but rejoices with the truth. It always protects, always trusts, always hopes, and always perseveres. Love never fails.
>
> 1 Corinthians 13:4–8 (NIV)

I want to thank my husband for sticking by me when things were bad and are still bad. So many of you have had your spouse walk out on you from having dysautonomia. I am so sorry for that, but try not to lose heart. God will never leave you. That is something you can truly rely on. Thank you, Ken, for your never-ending love and for accepting me just the way I am. Thank you for all the jobs you work and for all the times you stood in as Mom for our children. Kenneth and Tricia are successful today due in part to your love and hard work. God is well pleased with you, my dear husband.

Deadly Infection

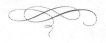

Dear friends do not be surprised at the painful trial you are suffering as though something strange were happening to you. But rejoice that you participate in the sufferings of Christ, so that you may be overjoyed when his glory is revealed.

1 Peter 4:12–13 (NIV)

On February 14, 2008, I was so ill that I couldn't move, breathe, or stand. I was shaking uncontrollably with a high fever. Ken called an ambulance to take me to the hospital. When I arrived, they rushed me to the ICU and called in a team of doctors. I had a bacterial infection. My liver and kidneys had stopped working, which is called renal failure. My bone marrow was eating itself, and my platelets were low. I couldn't breathe. I felt like death. Every breath I took was a struggle. I was so yellow and swollen I couldn't even lie on my side. They told my family to plan for the worst because people usually do not get over what my body was going through. Tricia came to see me daily. I didn't want people to come see me because I looked so bad and felt like death. On one visit my daughter told me not to leave her, that she needed me. People were praying from everywhere with prayer chains and meetings. I was so miserable I wanted to die just so the pain would go away.

"Dear Lord, it would be easy to die and be with you in heaven, but if you want me on earth as a sacrifice for you, then comfort me. Be my strength to fight this terrible infection. Help me, Lord. My hope is in you. Amen."

God and I spent night and day together. He showed me scriptures and comforted me. I was on oxygen, and every breath was torture. I gasped and gasped. I knew God was with me, right by my side, giving me peace. If I didn't have God's strength, I would not have made it through such a deadly infection. Because of how bad I felt, I kept wishing they would put me under, give me medicine to be out of it.

> But, those who suffer he delivers in their suffering, he speaks to them in their affliction.
>
> Job 36:15, NIV

> I will be glad and rejoice in your love, for you saw my affliction and knew the anguish of my soul.
>
> Psalm 1:7, NIV

Remember your word to your servant, for you have given me hope. My comfort in my suffering is this: Your promise preserves my life.

Psalm 119, NIV

Surely it was for my benefit that I suffered such anguish. In your love you kept me from the pit of destruction, you have put all my sins behind my back.

Isaiah 38:17, NIV

I prayed, "Thank you, Jesus, for dying on the cross to save me from my sins. It hurts to think that you suffered so badly, for I now understand through my suffering how terrible it must have been for you. Suffering with the infection was so hard, and I felt so terrible. I can't even fathom how you must have been hurting while you were on that cross." While I lay there unable to move, God spoke to me. I thought of my life and the past several years. When you are on your deathbed, *things* do not matter. Your looks, your hair, your clothes—none of that matters. At that horrible time I could only think of what I had done for God in my life. Had I shared Jesus as much as I could? As I lay in the hospital bed wondering if I would live, I could see hands stretched out and up toward heaven on my behalf. I saw little hands, young hands, old hands—all kinds were praying on my behalf. I was so sick. Was it a dream, or did God send that image to me? It did comfort me. And it was true; so many different types of people were praying for me.

Late one night, most of the lights were off, and the visiting hours were over, but I could see a figure coming through the door. When he came into the room, he knelt beside my bed and said, "Lynn, God has laid it on my heart to come and pray with you and to anoint your head with oil like the Bible says." I could feel his head as he knelt down beside my bed. It was Cade, one of the ministers from my church. He said, "The Bible didn't tell me what kind of oil to use, whether Crisco or what, so I just brought some we had in the house." He opened the oil and put it on my head and prayed one of the most heartfelt prayers I have ever heard. He pleaded with God, he gave my weak, sick body to God, and he asked God to heal me so I could be with my family. As he wept, I wept too. It meant so much, and I could feel God's touch while he was praying. I could tell his prayers were working throughout my body.

The next day things started working and improving. My kidneys were working. My liver was better. My blood work was also better. It was a miracle. Cade came to see me a few days later, and I was in the rehabilitation part of the hospital getting stronger. He shared with me how he had anointed my head with bath and body oil. He laughed when I told him that it smelled like lavender. It was so joyous to feel God's presence working in my body. I knew God must have a mighty plan for my life because I had pulled through that horrible infection.

But as for me, I will always have hope; I will
praise you more and more. My mouth will tell of
your righteousness, of your salvation all day long,
though I know not its measure. I will proclaim
your mighty acts, Oh Sovereign Lord; I will proclaim your righteousness, yours alone ... Though
you have made me see troubles, many and bitter,
you will restore my life again; from the depths
of the earth you will again bring me up. You will
increase my honor and comfort me once again.

Psalm 71:14–16, 20–21, NIV

I am glad my hope is in the Lord, and I will tell
of his righteousness and his mighty acts. God has
made me see so many troubles—some horrible—but
he always came to me wherever I was, which at times
felt like the end of the earth. God brought me up and
increased my comfort.

I always knew God wanted me to write a book
to tell of my journey, but I never knew when. After
coming close to dying, I knew one reason he healed
me from the infection was so I could write a book to
help others, to share God's miracles.

It is 2009, and I am still very ill. I suffer from
profound dysautonomia, a hole in my heart, mitral
valve prolapse, a hernia, acid reflux disease, deep vein
thrombosis, blood clots, hypothyroidism, anemia,
narrowing of the channel of the spine, degeneration
of the cervical and lumbar discs, seizures, myalgia,
and constant infections. I feel bad from the time I
get up in the morning until I go to bed at night. I
struggle daily to take care of myself, giving myself

IVs, medication, and shots. But what I do not suffer from is a lack of God's love, peace, and joy. God is my best friend.

I praise God because he has enabled me to serve in a way I never dreamed possible. He truly is a God of miracles—all kinds, great and small. Once I spent time with God and got closer to him, then I felt his wonderful love, and I knew it was better than life itself. I know this because he has shown me time and time again that through it all, God needs me for his kingdom.

"Because your love is better than life, my lips will glorify you" (Psalm 63:3, NIV).

God's love is like a little sprinkle of heaven. I have the best job in the world because God needs me.

A Personal Invitation

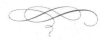

If after reading *God Needs Me,* you realize that you have never accepted the salvation of Jesus, you can receive this salvation. I invite you to receive him right now. In Christ is total forgiveness of sins, total acceptance, love, and eternal life.

> For God so loved the world that He gave his one and only Son, that whoever believes in Him shall not perish but have eternal life. For God did not send His Son into the world to condemn the world but to save the world through him.
>
> John 3:16–17, NIV

Dear Heavenly Father,

I know I am a sinner. You sent Jesus Christ into the world to save me. He died on a cross so my sins would be forgiven. Jesus Christ rose from the grave, and I believe in him. By accepting Jesus Christ into my heart, I will live eternally in heaven when I die here on earth. The only way is through Jesus. I am accepting Jesus Christ as my Savior right now. Jesus, forgive me for my sins. I am asking you into my heart. I want to learn how to lean totally on you for every aspect of my life. In you is total forgiveness of sins, total acceptance, love, and eternal life.

In Jesus Christ's name,
Amen.

If you are already saved but after reading *God Needs Me,* you have discovered that you do not have a personal relationship with God, you can pray for that.

Dear Heavenly Father,

I have already accepted Jesus Christ into my heart. But Lord, I want you for my best friend. I want you to shower me with your love, peace, and joy. I will spend more time telling you how much I love you. I will spend more time in your Word. Then I will know the things you have planned for me in my life. I realize that I am here on earth for you, Lord, and not for myself, whether sick or well. I will share you with others in need. I am asking you to help me learn to draw closer to you. I am going to rely on you for my strength, instead of myself or others, because you can do anything. Please forgive me for not loving you enough and for not sharing you with others in need. Thank you, Lord, for all the blessings of my life. I want to work for you because you need me.

In Jesus Christ's name,
Amen.